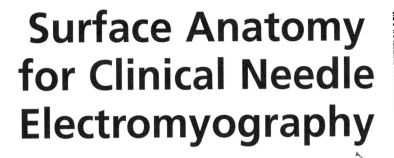

Surface Anatomy for Clinical Needle Electromyography

Hang J. Lee, M.D.

*Professor, Department of Rehabilitation Medicine
Korea University College of Medicine, Seoul, Korea*

*Formerly Associate Professor, Presently Visiting Associate Professor,
Department of Physical Medicine and Rehabilitation,
UMDNJ–New Jersey Medical School,
Newark, New Jersey*

AND

Joel A. DeLisa, M.D., M.S.

*Professor and Chairman, Department of Physical Medicine
and Rehabilitation, UMDNJ–New Jersey Medical School,
Newark, New Jersey*

*President, Kessler Medical Rehabilitation Research
and Education Corporation, West Orange, New Jersey*

*Senior Vice-President and Chief Medical Officer,
Kessler Rehabilitation Corporation,
West Orange, New Jersey*

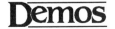

Demos

Demos Medical Publishing, Inc., 386 Park Avenue South, New York, New York 10016

Library of Congress Cataloging-in-Publication Data

Available from the publisher upon request

Made in the United States of America

DEDICATION

To Young Lee, Hang Lee's wife,
and to his children, Edward and Jennifer Lee

To the memory of Alice DeLisa, Joel DeLisa's mother,
for her insistence on her children attending college and instilling in
them a work ethic

Contents

THE HAND

THE FOREARM

THE ARM

THE SHOULDER

THE FOOT

THE LEG

THE ANTERIOR THIGH

THE BUTTOCK AND POSTERIOR THIGH

THE TRUNK

THE PELVIS

THE HEAD AND NECK

Preface

This manual was designed to be used by physicians in electrodiagnosis training and electromyographers in practice to help identify and localize specific skeletal muscles they want to study. The manual was developed for use in the electrodiagnosis laboratory and is not intended to replace standard textbooks and reference literature.

This manual is divided into 12 sections: hand, forearm, arm, shoulder, foot, leg, anterior thigh, buttock and posterior thigh, trunk (chest, abdomen), back, pelvis, and head and neck.

Each muscle in each section has the following format: patient position, needle (electrode insertion), clinical notes, innervation, origin, and insertion. This is followed by an illustration that highlights clinical landmarks to aid in the needle electrode location.

Although there usually is more than one method of inserting the needle into the muscle that you wish to study, the authors have indicated their preferences.

The authors hope that this manual will be a useful and practical edition to be used along with their *Manual of Nerve Conduction Velocity and Clinical Neurophysiology.*

We welcome your critique and suggestions.

Introduction

A well-planned needle EMG examination and the patient's cooperation are critical for an optimal study for:

1. Minimizing the number of needle penetrations
2. Minimizing the patient's discomfort
3. Shortening the length of the examination
4. Obtaining the maximal information toward the diagnosis

A complete successful needle electrode examination includes:

A. History and physical examination:

1. Review the patient's history and diagnostic workup.
2. Perform a brief focused physical examination of the neuromuscular and musculoskeletal system.

B. Reducing the anxiety and fear of needling and/or electrical shock

1. Explain the various portions of the procedure using very simple language.

Some patients are very apprehensive and expect (have been told) that the test will hurt. Patients with less fear and anxiety will be able to cooperate better and the electromyographer will obtain all the necessary information.

2. Explain that you will be using a very fine disposable needle (with the exception of SFEMG needles, which are nondisposable).
3. No electric current or stimuli will be given through the needle.
4. No injection will be given through the needle.
5. Explain that the sound is coming from the muscle activity and is an intricate part of the examination.
6. Explain that you will test only a sufficient number of muscles to make a diagnosis.

C. Patient position: Find the most comfortable position on the examination table or chair to ensure the patient's cooperation. Possible positions are:

1. Supine-lying
2. Lateral decubitus (side-lying): fetal position (full flexion of neck, trunk, hips and knees) is very helpful for full relaxation of the paraspinal muscles.
3. Prone position (to support and relax the testing areas, pillows are placed at various parts of the body: neck, chest, abdomen, hip, knee, ankle, etc.)
4. Sitting

Place the patient in the most comfortable position on the examination table, with the site of the needle insertion visible and within easy reach of the examiner. The patient, examiner and EMG machine must be in close proximity.

D. Preparation of studying areas

1. Expose the area to be studied.
2. Clean the skin with alcohol in all areas to be tested. Wait for the alcohol to evaporate before inserting the needle. Needling on an area of skin wet from alcohol is quite painful (burning sensation).
3. If the room is cold, cover the exposed limb or trunk for the patient's comfort.

E. Identification of the muscle to be tested using the landmarks:

1. Origin and insertion point of the muscle
2. Palpation of the muscle belly or tendon movement of activation of the muscle to be tested
3. Bones and their landmarks
4. Boundary of the adjacent muscles
5. Artery and its pulse

It is necessary to be familiar with surface and functional anatomy before insertion of the needle into the muscle. To confirm the proper needle placement, the patient may be asked to activate the testing muscle. However, this procedure may not be possible in patients with severe motor axonal loss. The deep muscles, e.g., tibialis posterior, flexor digitorum profundus, diaphragm (also refer to text), are very difficult to identify, but our labeled drawings and descriptions should be helpful.

F. Order of muscle sampling on needle exam:

1. Proximal to distal in the limb as the proximal muscles are usually less sensitive to needle insertion than the distal small muscles.

2. The weakest muscle and greatest probability for revealing abnormalities may be tested first (more abnormal muscle first in the anxious patient or children). However, the end stage of muscle pathology may not give findings and that must be interpreted carefully.

3. The less painful muscle should be examined first. Intrinsic muscles of the hands and feet are usually very painful.

4. Some patients prefer needle EMG rather than the shocks associated with nerve conduction studies.

5. Consult an expert if you are to study unfamiliar muscles and prepare well before the examination, taking the necessary precautions.

G. Avoid needle penetration through the following organs if possible:

1. Major vessels—arteries and veins

2. Excretory glands

3. Nerves

4. Tendons

5. Viscera

6. Infection sites

7. Ulcer areas

8. Scar

9. Edema, including lymphedema

H. During the needle insertion:

1. Hold the needle firmly by the thumb and fingers.

2. Make the needle insertion skin site taut by the thumb and fingers (e.g., biceps or gastrocnemius).

3. Insert the needle through the skin at a perpendicular angle (large and thick muscle) or sharp angle (thin layer of muscle). Needle insertion by quick thrust is less painful.

Concentric needle—initially insert the needle at a perpendicular angle (directly to the skin or muscle in large muscle), but parallel to the muscle fibers (monopolar needle also). For thin layered muscle, insert at a sharp angle (facial muscles).

An extra-long (75 mm) needle is necessary for the very obese patient.

4. Guide the path of the needle into the muscle with your fingers to avoid puncturing the viscera, e.g. serratus anterior, rhomboid, trapezius, orbicularis oculi, etc. Extra precaution is necessary: near the visceral muscles in the neck, chest-thoracic wall (pneumothorax), neck and abdominal wall muscles.

5. Move the needle 2 to 3 mm in each step to check insertional/spontaneous activities and to reduce pain.

6. To look for spontaneous activities, pause a few seconds after each needle movement in the muscle.

7. To reduce pain, avoid needle insertion if possible in the following areas: endplate region, nerve, tendon, periosteum, etc.

8. A needle penetration through the skin, subcutaneous tissue, and muscle should include more than five insertions in a straight line depending on the depth (thickness) of the muscle. Withdraw the needle tip, placing it under the subcutaneous tissue or skin and reinsert in a different direction.

9. Check the needle insertion site for bleeding, oozing, leakage of edematous fluid, or a bruise. A firm pressure with dried cotton balls or sterilized 2" x 2" gauze may be necessary.

I. Special precautions—diseases/problems:

1. Infection—HIV positive, viral hepatitis, Creutzfeldt-Jacob disease
   - Use disposable needles.
   - Wear disposable gloves, mask, goggles, and plastic gowns to prevent these transmissible diseases.
   - Pay attention to areas that are unavoidable to touch, e.g., EMG keyboard, needle connector, extension wires, preamplifier, etc., when your hands are contaminated with blood or body fluid during the test. Clean the contaminated equipment with proper disinfectants (refer to the manufacturer's manual).
   - Clean the items contaminated with blood or body fluid with the proper concentration of bleach.
   - Tongue or anal sphincter muscles should be tested last.

2. Bleeding disorders—hemophilia, anticoagulant therapy, thrombocytopenia

3. Rheumatic heart disease, valvular heart disease with prosthetic valves—risk of bacterial endocarditis or transient bacteremia

4. Extreme obesity—difficult to identify the location of the muscle, e.g. most of the chest or thoracic, abdominal wall muscles, diaphragm, etc.

To get all the necessary information for the electrophysiologic diagnosis, any available muscle can be chosen for needle examination. Some muscles are more frequently tested than others. Noted below are the muscles that appeared as case reports or minimonographs in the journal *Muscle & Nerve* during the last 10 years. However, this does not mean that these muscles are more important than other muscles.

supraspinatus

infraspinatus

pectoralis major

rhomboid

trapezius

deltoid

biceps

triceps—long head and lateral head

pronator teres

flexor carpi radialis

flexor carpi ulnaris

abductor digiti minimi

first dorsal interosseous

abductor pollicis brevis

extensor digitorum communis

extensor carpi ulnaris

extensor indicis

flexor pollicis longus

flexor digitorum superficialis

flexor digitorum profundus (radial side)

opponens pollicis

pronator quadratus

serratus anterior

paraspinous muscle-high cervicals and low cervicals

thoracic paraspinals

lumbar paraspinals (by L4 and 5)

tibialis anterior

gastrocnemius (medial and lateral)

vastus medialis

vastus lateralis

tensor fascia lata

semitendinosus

semimembranosus

gluteus maximus

gluteus medius

biceps femoris-short head

tibialis posterior

abductor hallucus brevis

flexor digitorum longus

abductor digiti quinti
extensor hallicus longus
rectus orbicularis oris
masseter
mentalis
orbicularis oculi
tongue
diaphragm
frontalis

References

Stevens JC. 1995 AAEEM Courses D: Practical suggestions for performing the needle electrode examination. pp. 27–32

Capozzoli NJ. Aseptic technique in needle EMG: Common sense and common practice. *Muscle & Nerve* 1996:19;538.

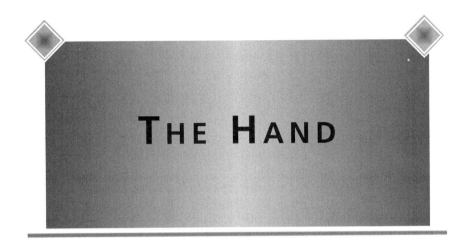

THE HAND

1. Abductor Pollicis Brevis

Patient position: Forearm supinated with the palm up

Needle insertion: Insert the needle obliquely from the radial side of the thenar eminence at about the proximal half of the first metacarpal bone.

Activation: Abduct the thumb with some medial rotation.

Clinical notes: If inserted too medially in the thenar eminence, the needle will penetrate the flexor pollicis brevis (superficial or deep head); if too deep, the opponens pollicis will be penetrated. It is thin and is the most superficial and lateral of the thenar muscles. In severe median neuropathy, a needle recording from this muscle may not eliminate the volume-conducted response from adjacent ulnar nerve innervated muscles. This muscle is very painful on needling!

Innervation: C8, T1—lower trunk—medial cord—median nerve (recurrent branch)

Origin: Flexor retinaculum, scaphoid, trapezium

Insertion: Radial (lateral) side of the base of the proximal phalanx of the thumb, and lateral sesamoid bone of the thumb

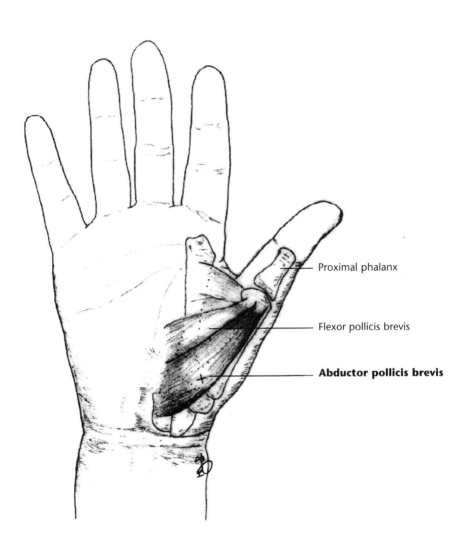

Proximal phalanx

Flexor pollicis brevis

Abductor pollicis brevis

2. Opponens Pollicis

Patient position: Forearm supinated with palm up

Needle insertion: This muscle is deep to the abductor pollicis brevis in the thenar eminence. Insert the needle close to the anterior surface of the first metacarpal bone.

Activation: Opposition of the thumb or flexion of the metacarpal bone of the thumb

Clinical notes: It is found deep to the abductor pollicis brevis. Atrophy is noted by flatness of the thenar eminence. It may occasionally be innervated by the deep branch of the ulnar nerve.

Innervation: C8, T1—lower trunk—medial cord—median nerve (recurrent branch)

Origin: Flexor retinaculum and trapezium

Insertion: Entire lateral border of the first metacarpal bone

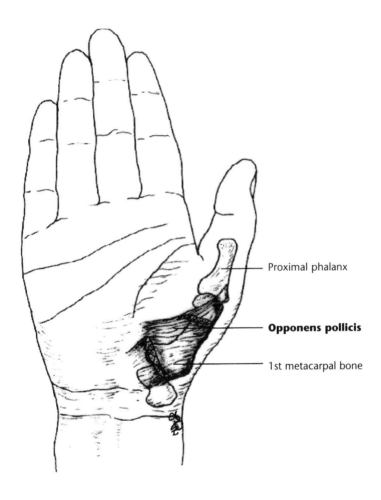

Proximal phalanx

Opponens pollicis

1st metacarpal bone

3. Flexor Pollicis Brevis—Superficial and Deep Head

Patient position: Supine with the forearm supinated and palm up

Needle insertion: Thenar eminence can be divided into lateral and medial halves by a longitudinal section. Insert the needle into the medial half area of the thenar eminence.

Activation: Flex the thumb (proximal phalanx); it also aids opposition and adduction.

Clinical notes: This muscle is found medial to the abductor pollicis brevis and is somewhat overlapped by it. It is particularly active in firm grip between the thumb, index and middle fingers.

Innervation: C8, T1—Superficial head: median nerve (recurrent branch) Deep head: ulnar nerve

Origin: Superficial head: Flexor retinaculum, trapezium and trapezoid Deep head: volar surfaces of the second and third metacarpals

Insertion: Radial (lateral) side of the base of the proximal phalanx of the thumb (medial to the insertion of the abductor pollicis brevis)

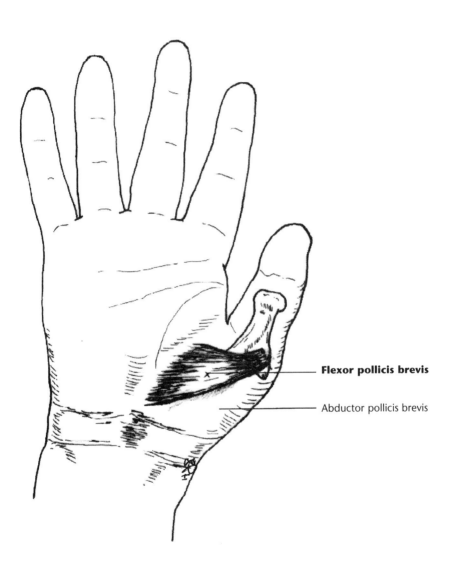

Flexor pollicis brevis

Abductor pollicis brevis

4. Lumbricals/First Lumbrical

Patient position: Palm up (supinated)

Needle insertion: Insert the needle at the radial side just proximal to the second metacarpophalangeal (MP) joint. This site is more preferable than the other three lumbricals.

Activation: Extend the interphalangeal (IP) joint of the second, third, fourth and fifth digits; flex the MP joint.

Innervation: The first and second lumbricals are innervated by the median nerve (C8, T1), while the third and fourth are supplied by the deep branch of the ulnar nerve (C8, T1).

Clinical notes: These are small cylindrical muscles of the palm of the hand. If inserted too deeply and proximally on examination of the first lumbrical, it will enter either the adductor pollicis or the first dorsal interosseous.

Origin: Tendons of flexor digitorum profundus

Insertion: Lateral margin of dorsal digital expansion at proximal phalangeal level, more distal than the interossei

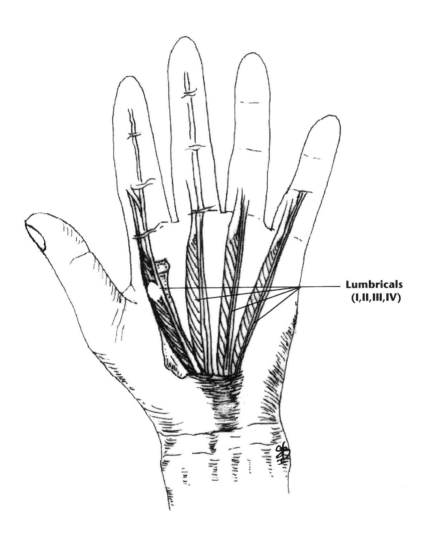

Lumbricals (I,II,III,IV)

5. First Dorsal Interosseous (Hand)

Patient position: Forearm and hand in a position halfway between supination and pronation

Needle insertion: Insert the needle at the center (most prominent belly of this muscle) of the dorsal first web space. If inserted too deeply, it will be in the adductor pollicis.

Clinical note: Three percent to ten percent of the population have median nerve innervation of the first dorsal interosseous. The first dorsal interosseous is larger than the others.

Activation: Abduct the second digit.

Innervation: C8, T1—lower trunk—anterior division—medial cord—ulnar nerve (deep branch)

Origin: **Lateral head**—from the dorsal surface of the proximal half of the ulnar border of the first metacarpal bone

Medial head—dorsal surface of the radial border of the second metacarpal bone

Insertion: Radial side of the proximal phalanx of the second digit, and the radial side lateral bands of the second extensor tendon hood

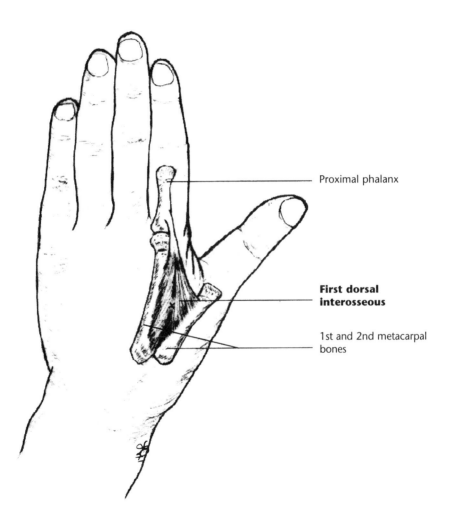

Proximal phalanx

First dorsal interosseous

1st and 2nd metacarpal bones

6. Adductor Pollicis

Patient position: Hand and forearm in the mid-half position

Needle insertion: Insert the needle at the distal half of the ulnar border of the first metacarpal bone obliquely toward the palm and the second metacarpal bone.

Activation: Adduct the thumb.

Clinical notes: If the needle is advanced too medially, it will be in the first dorsal interosseous. It lies deep in the palm in contact with the metacarpals and the interossei muscles.

Innervation: C8, T1—lower trunk—anterior division—medial cord—ulnar nerve (deep branch). Infrequently it is innervated by the median nerve.

Origin: The second and third metacarpal bones, and the capitate and trapezoid bones

Insertion: Medial side of the base of the proximal phalanx of the thumb and the medial sesamoid bone of the thumb. Also the extensor tendon of the extensor pollicis longus

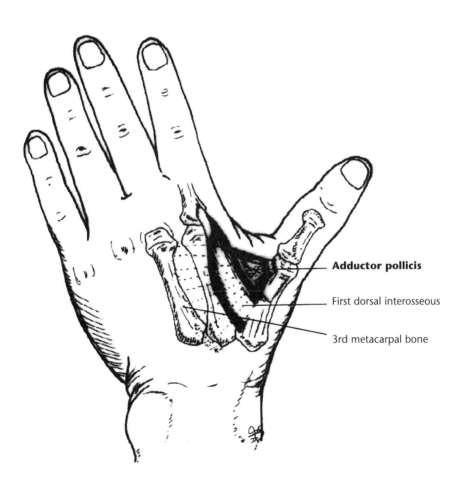

Adductor pollicis

First dorsal interosseous

3rd metacarpal bone

7. First Palmar Interosseous

Patient position: Palm up

Needle insertion: Insert the needle at the ulnar side of the mid-half of the second metacarpal bone.

Activation: Adduct the second digit to the third digit.

Clinical note: The line of reference with respect to abductor or adductor in the hand is the middle finger.

Innervation: C8, T1—lower trunk—medial cord—ulnar nerve (deep branch)

Origin: Entire ulnar side of the palmar surface of the second metacarpal bone

Insertion: Same side of the digital expansion of the index finger

Base of the proximal phalanx of the index finger

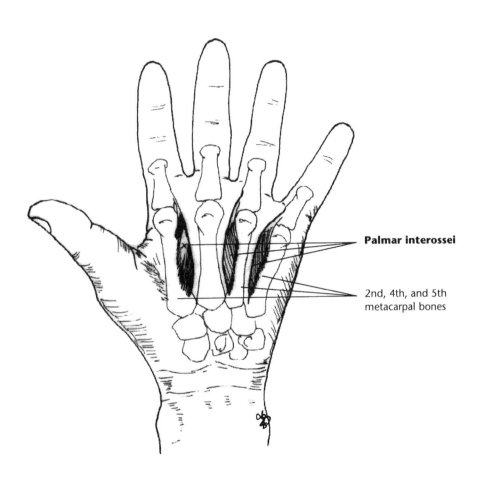

Palmar interossei

2nd, 4th, and 5th
metacarpal bones

8. Abductor Digiti Minimi

Patient position: Forearm supinated with the palm up or forearm pronated with the palm down

Needle insertion: Insert the needle from the ulnar aspect of the hand at about the proximal one-third point between the distal wrist crease and the proximal digital crease.

Activation: Abduct the little finger away from the ring finger, with flexion of the proximal phalanx at the metacarpophalangeal joint.

Clinical notes: It is the most superficial and medial of the hypothenar muscles. It forms the ulnar convex surface of the hand.

Innervation: C8, T1—lower trunk—medial cord—ulnar nerve (deep branch)

Origin: Pisiform bone and tendon of flexor carpi ulnaris

Insertion: Ulnar (medial) side of the base of the proximal phalanx of the fifth digit

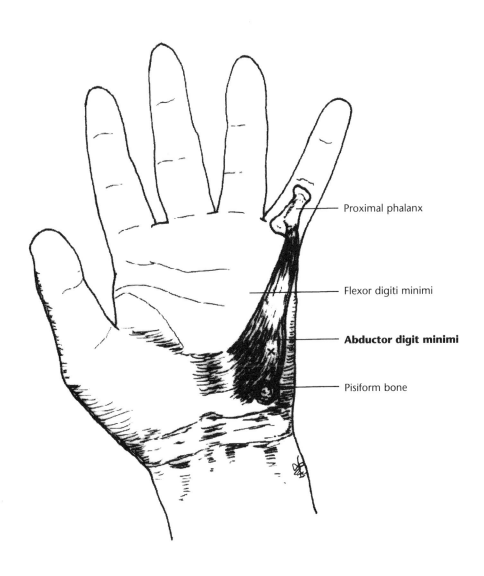

Proximal phalanx

Flexor digiti minimi

Abductor digit minimi

Pisiform bone

9. Flexor Digiti Minimi Brevis

Patient position: Supine with palm up

Needle insertion: Insert the needle at the midpoint between the proximal digital crease of the fifth finger and distal wrist crease.

Activation: Flex the fifth finger at the metacarpophalangeal joint.

Clinical notes: The muscle lies on the radial (lateral) side of the abductor digiti minimi and may be missing. It is the most superficial of the hypothenar muscles.

Innervation: C8, T1—lower trunk—medial cord—ulnar nerve (deep branch)

Origin: Hook of the hamate bone and the palmar surface of the flexor retinaculum

Insertion: Ulnar side of the base of the proximal phalanx of the fifth digit

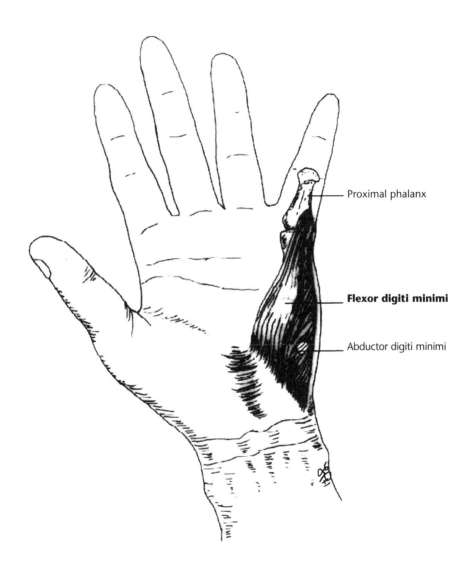

Proximal phalanx

Flexor digiti minimi

Abductor digiti minimi

10. Opponens Digiti Minimi

Patient position: Supine with the forearm supinated and the palm up

Needle insertion: This muscle lies deep to the abductor digiti minimi (ADM) and partly covers the fifth metacarpal bone in the volar aspect of the palm. Insert the needle at the mid-half of the fifth metacarpal bone from the ulnar side. The needle is inserted close to the bone in the palm side and advanced radially in the coronal plane. While advancing, the ADM is pushed radially.

Activation: Opposition of the fifth finger to the thumb

Innervation: C8, T1—lower trunk—medial cord—ulnar nerve

Origin: Hook of hamate and flexor retinaculum

Insertion: Entire length of the ulnar margin of the front of the fifth metacarpal bone

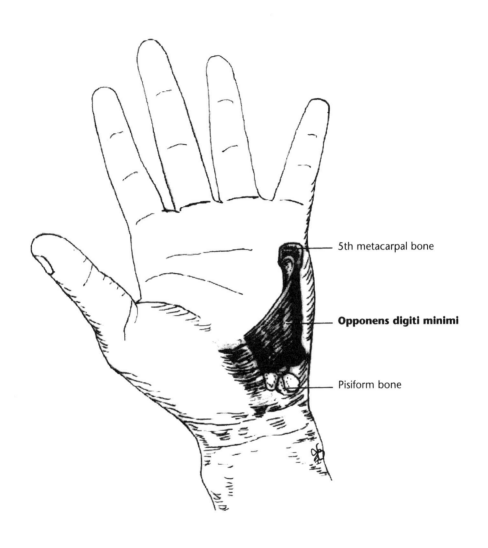

5th metacarpal bone

Opponens digiti minimi

Pisiform bone

THE FOREARM

11. Pronator Teres

Patient position:	Supine with the forearm supinated
Needle insertion:	Place the index finger on the cubital fossa and insert the needle medially to the finger at approximately 5 cm below the elbow crease.
Activation:	Pronate the forearm with the slight elbow flexion
Clinical notes:	The ulnar head of the pronator teres is congenitally absent in approximately 9% of the population. The pronator teres is the uppermost member of the forearm flexors, and it passes obliquely across the forearm. If inserted too deeply, the needle may penetrate the median nerve or brachial artery; too medially, the flexor carpi radialis. The median nerve passes between the two heads of origin and may become entrapped.
Innervation:	C6, 7—upper and middle trunk—anterior division—lateral cord—median nerve
Origin:	Medial epicondyle of the humerus by a common flexor tendon and coronoid process of the ulnar
Insertion:	Lateral surface of the radius to the midline (wraps around the radius)

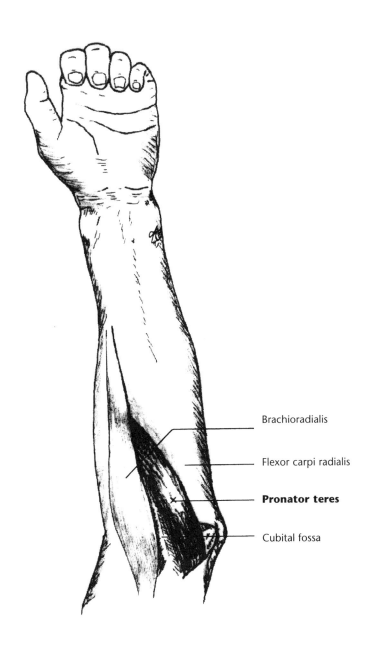

Brachioradialis

Flexor carpi radialis

Pronator teres

Cubital fossa

12. Flexor Carpi Radialis

Patient position: Supine with forearm supinated

Needle insertion: Insert the needle at a distance of one-third or one-half proximally between the tendon of flexor carpi radialis at the wrist and the medial supracondylar area of humerus.

Activation: Flex and abduct the wrist (radial deviation).

Clinical notes: It is medial to the pronator teres. It is a superficial muscle and is not clearly demarcated from the adjacent muscles. At the wrist this median nerve lies medial to the tendon of the flexor carpi radialis. This muscle may be involved in the pronator syndrome. If the needle is inserted too laterally, it will be in the pronator teres; too medially, it will be in the palmaris longus; too deeply, it will be in the flexor digitorum superficialis or flexor digitorum profundus.

Innervation: C6, C7—median nerve

Origin: Medial epicondyle of the humerus by a common flexor tendon

Insertion: Base of the volar surface of the second metacarpal bone. It frequently also inserts into the scaphoid bone.

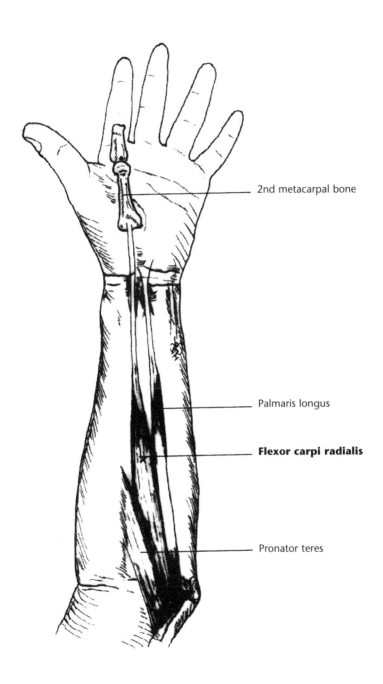

2nd metacarpal bone

Palmaris longus

Flexor carpi radialis

Pronator teres

13. Palmaris Longus

Patient position: Supine with the forearm fully supinated

Needle insertion: Insert the needle at the proximal upper third of a line drawn between the palmaris longus tendon at the wrist crease and medial epicondyle of the humerus.

Activation: Flex the wrist.

Clinical notes: The muscle is superficial, slender, fusiform, and medial to the flexor carpi radialis. If inserted too deeply, it will be the flexor digitorum superficialis. This muscle is absent in approximately 10–15% of the population and is subject to a lot of variation. The tendon can be demonstrated by opposing the thumb to the little finger against resistance.

Innervation: C7, C8—median nerve

Origin: Medial epicondyle of the humerus by a common tendon

Insertion: Palmar aponeurosis and flexor retinaculum

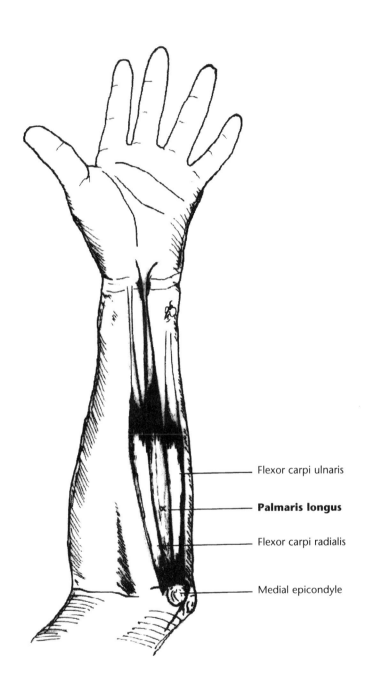

Flexor carpi ulnaris

Palmaris longus

Flexor carpi radialis

Medial epicondyle

14. Flexor Digitorum Superficialis (Sublimis)

Patient position: Supine with the forearm supinated

Needle insertion: Identify the tendons of palmaris longus and flexor carpi ulnaris at the wrist and follow proximally to the mid-forearm where the needle is inserted. The muscle is more superficial at this point.

Activation: Flex the middle phalanx of each of the medial four digits.

Clinical notes: If the needle is inserted too deeply, it will be in the flexor digitorum profundus. Entrapment of the anterior interosseous nerve occurs by either a fibrous origin of this muscle or a tendinous origin of it to the third digit.

Innervation: C7, C8, and T1—median nerve

Origin: Medial epicondyle of the humerus by a common flexor tendon, coronoid process of the ulna, and ulnar collateral ligament of the elbow joint. Also from the oblique line of the anterior radius below the radial tuberosity.

Insertion: This muscle divides into four tendons above the wrist and inserts into the palmar aspect of the middle phalanx of the medial four digits.

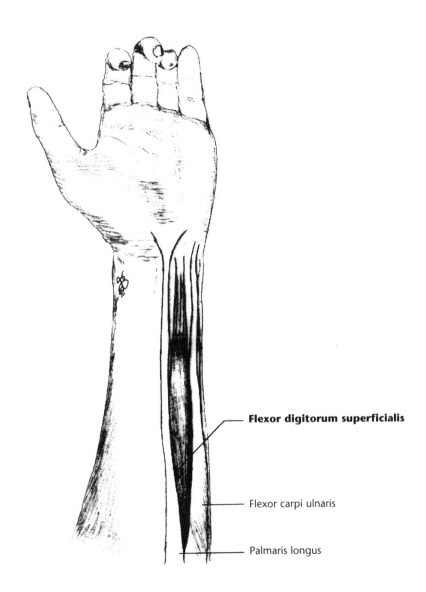

Flexor digitorum superficialis

Flexor carpi ulnaris

Palmaris longus

15. Flexor Pollicis Longus

Patient position: Supine with forearm supinated

Needle insertion: Insert the needle at the junction of the middle and distal third of the forearm between the brachioradialis and flexor carpi radialis. Before inserting, note the radial pulse at the insertion site.

Activation: Flex the distal phalanx of the thumb.

Clinical notes: It is the only muscle that flexes the interphalangeal joint of the thumb. In the diagnostic work-up of carpal tunnel syndrome, this muscle is examined to rule out the possibility of a more proximal involvement of the median nerve.

innervation: C8 and T1—lower trunk—medial cord— anterior interosseous branch (nerve) of the median nerve

Origin: Anterior surface of the middle half of the radius, adjoining anterior interosseous membrane and deep fascia

Insertion: Base of the volar surface of the distal phalanx of the thumb

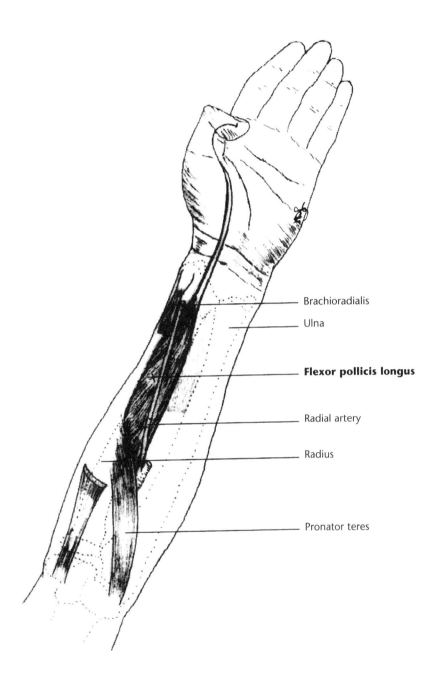

Brachioradialis

Ulna

Flexor pollicis longus

Radial artery

Radius

Pronator teres

16. Pronator Quadratus

Patient position:	Supine with forearm supinated or pronated
Needle insertion:	**1.** From the ulnar (medial) side of the forearm, insert the needle close to the anterior surface of the ulna, 2 to 3 cm proximal to the ulnar styloid. On insertion, put a finger under the tendon of flexor carpi ulnaris and push it to the radial side.
	2. Identify a cleft between the layers of extensor tendons over the dorsal aspect of the distal forearm (distal fourth between the lateral epicondyle and ulnar styloid). Insert the needle between tendons and supinate forearm into the neutral position and slowly advance it through the interosseous membrane and finally into the pronator quadratus.*
Clinical notes:	This is the most distal muscle innervated by the anterior interosseous nerve. This is one of the deepest muscles of the forearm flexor muscles and is flat and quadrilateral in shape. It is examined for a conduction study of the anterior interosseous nerve.
Innervation:	C8, T1—lower trunk—medial cord—median nerve (anterior interosseous nerve)
Origin:	Anteromedial aspect, distal quarter of the ulna
Insertion:	Anteromedial border, distal quarter of the radius
	*(*Reference:* Wertsch JJ: AAEM case report #25: Anterior interosseous nerve syndrome. *Muscle & Nerve* 15: 977–983, 1992)

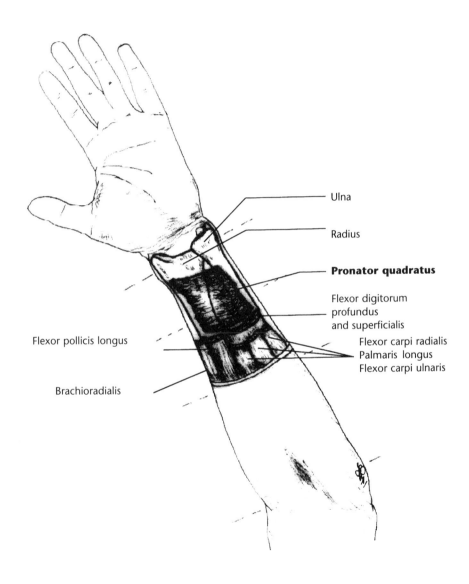

Ulna

Radius

Pronator quadratus

Flexor digitorum
profundus
and superficialis

Flexor carpi radialis
Palmaris longus
Flexor carpi ulnaris

Flexor pollicis longus

Brachioradialis

17. Flexor Carpi Ulnaris

Patient position: Supine and forearm supinated

Needle insertion: Insert the needle at the mid-third of a line drawn between the ulnar styloid and medial epicondyle. When supinated, this muscle is most medially located. If the needle is inserted too deeply, it will pass into either the flexor digitorum sublimis or profundus.

Activation:
1. Flex and abduct (ulnar deviation) the wrist or simply flex and abduct the fifth digit.
2. Abduct the fifth digit without wrist flexion.*

Clinical notes: This is the only muscle to insert into a carpal bone. In ulnar nerve compression at the elbow, this muscle is often spared.

Innervation: C8, T1—lower trunk—medial cord—ulnar nerve

Origin: Medial epicondyle of the humerus by a common tendon and the medial border of the olecranon process and the posterior border of the upper 3/5 the ulna.

Insertion: First into the pisiform bone, then to the hook of the hamate, and finally into the base of the fifth metacarpal by the piso-hamate and piso-metacarpal ligaments

*(Reference: Roberts MM, Wertsch JJ, Park TA, Mazur A, Oswald TA: Selective activation of the flexor carpi ulnaris. Muscle & Nerve 17: 1099, 1994)

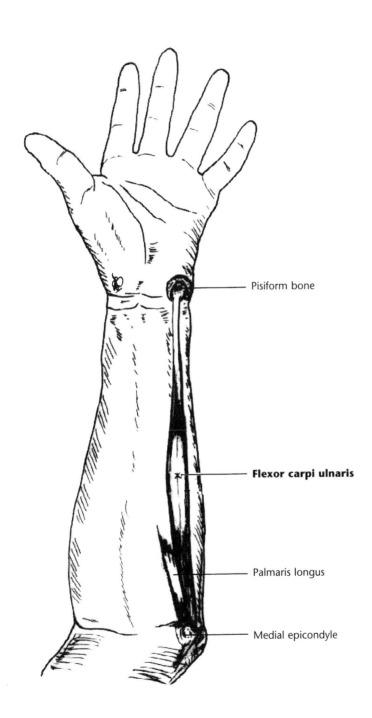

Pisiform bone

Flexor carpi ulnaris

Palmaris longus

Medial epicondyle

18. Flexor Digitorum Profundus

Patient position: Supine with elbow flexed and forearm fully pronated

Needle insertion: Insert the needle from the medial border at the middle third of the ulna and advance it tangentially toward the radial side, pushing the muscle belly of the flexor carpi ulnaris/flexor digitorum superficialis radially.

Activation: Flex the distal phalanx of the medial four digits.

Clinical notes: It is the bulkiest of the forearm muscles. This muscle has a dual innervation—the radial side by the median nerve and the ulnar side by the ulnar nerve. This is true in approximately 60% of cases. In the other 40%, the median and ulnar nerve distribution is 3: 1 or 1: 3 equally. Examine to verify the selective involvement of the anterior interosseous nerve or a branch of the ulnar nerve. Needle placement to this muscle is not easy anatomically or technically. It is preferable to use the other muscles such as the flexor pollicis longus or the pronator quadratus.

Innervation: C7–8 and T1—middle and lower trunk— anterior division— median (anterior interosseous nerve) and ulnar nerve

Origin: Proximal three-fourths of anterior surface of ulna, medial half of the anterior interosseous membrane and the deep fascia

Insertion: Palmar surface of the distal phalanx of each of the medial four digits

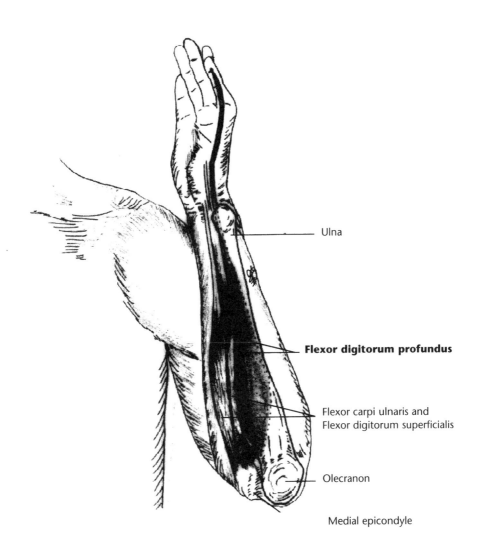

Ulna

Flexor digitorum profundus

Flexor carpi ulnaris and
Flexor digitorum superficialis

Olecranon

Medial epicondyle

19. Brachioradialis

Patient position: Supine with forearm supinated

Needle insertion: Identify the cubital fossa by placing the index finger at the elbow. The border of the fossa is formed by the brachioradialis laterally and pronator teres medially. Insert the needle approximately 1 cm laterally from the cubital fossa and 1 cm below the elbow crease with the forearm supinated.

Activation: Flex the elbow with the forearm supinated.

Clinical notes: Found superficial to the forearm extensors and is located on the anterolateral aspect of the arm. It is the most anterior of the forearm extensors. Radial neuropathy in the midhumerus or spiral groove usually shows abnormal EMG findings in the brachioradialis with the triceps spared. Therefore, this muscle is important to identify the localization of radial nerve lesion in a wrist drop.

Innervation: C5, C6—upper trunk—posterior division—posterior cord—radial nerve.

Origin: Lateral supracondylar ridge of the humerus and the lateral intermuscular septum

Insertion: Lateral aspect of the radial styloid process

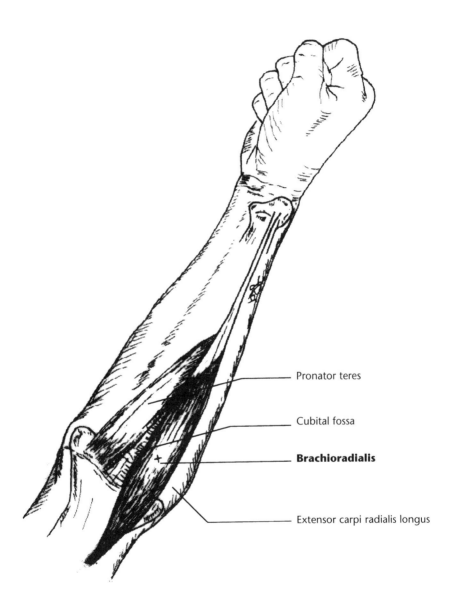

Pronator teres

Cubital fossa

Brachioradialis

Extensor carpi radialis longus

20. Extensor Carpi Radialis Longus and Brevis

Patient position: Supine with the forearm pronated

Needle insertion: *Longus:* With forearm fully pronated, the most prominent area radially just below the elbow is formed by this muscle. Insert the needle 2 to 3 cm distal to the elbow joint over the most prominent area of that muscle bulk.

Brevis: Insert the needle a little bit distal and just lateral to the extensor carpi radialis longus.

Activation: Extend and abduct the wrist, flex the elbow.

Clinical notes: After innervating the extensor carpi radialis brevis, the radial nerve becomes the posterior interosseous nerve that passes through the supinator.

Innervation: C6, 7—upper and middle trunk— posterior division—posterior cord—radial nerve

Extensor Carpi Radialis Longus:

Origin: Distal third of the lateral supracondylar ridge of the humerus and lateral intermuscular septum

Insertion: Dorsal surface, base of the second metacarpal bone

Extensor Carpi Radialis Brevis:

Origin: Lateral epicondyle of the humerus (common extensor tendon) and radial collateral ligament of the elbow joint

Insertion: Dorsal surface, base of the third metacarpal

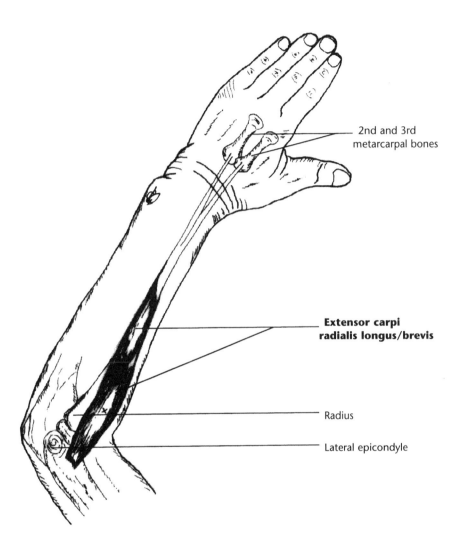

2nd and 3rd
metarcarpal bones

**Extensor carpi
radialis longus/brevis**

Radius

Lateral epicondyle

21. Extensor Carpi Ulnaris

Patient position: Supine with the forearm pronated

Needle insertion: Insert the needle at the midpoint between the lateral epicondyle of the humerus and the ulnar styloid.

Activation: Extend and adduct the hand or abduct and extend the fifth digit.

Innervation: C7, C8—middle and lower trunk—posterior division—posterior cord—radial nerve (posterior interosseous nerve)

Origin: Lateral epicondyle of the humerus by a common extensor tendon and posterior aspect of the ulna

Insertion: Dorsal surface of the base of the fifth metacarpal bone

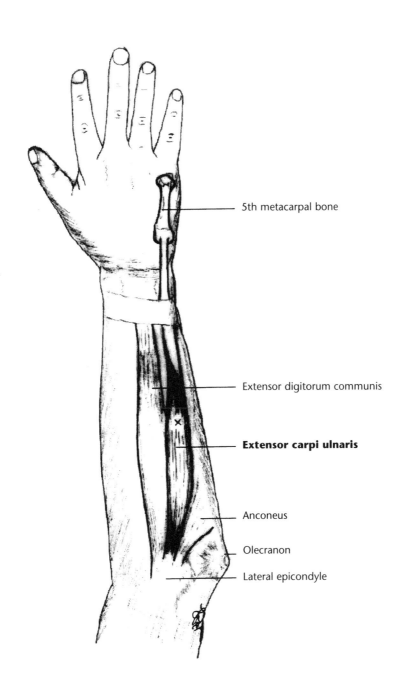

5th metacarpal bone

Extensor digitorum communis

Extensor carpi ulnaris

Anconeus

Olecranon

Lateral epicondyle

22. Extensor Digitorum Communis

Patient position: Supine with the forearm pronated

Needle insertion: Insert the needle at the upper third on a line drawn between the lateral epicondyle of the humerus and the midpoint of a line between the radial and ulnar styloid at the wrist.

Activation: Extend the second and third fingers.

Clinical notes: This muscle occupies much of the extensor surface of the forearm. Weakness of this muscle will result in a position of flexion of the proximal phalanges. This muscle is examined for single fiber electromyography.

Innervation: C7, C8—middle and lower trunk—posterior division—posterior cord—radial nerve (posterior interosseous nerve)

Origin: Lateral epicondyle of humerus by a common extensor tendon

Insertion: Divides into four tendons above the wrist and inserts into the extensor tendon hood with a central slip to the middle phalanx of 2, 3, 4, 5 and two collateral slips to the terminal phalanx of 2, 3, 4, 5.

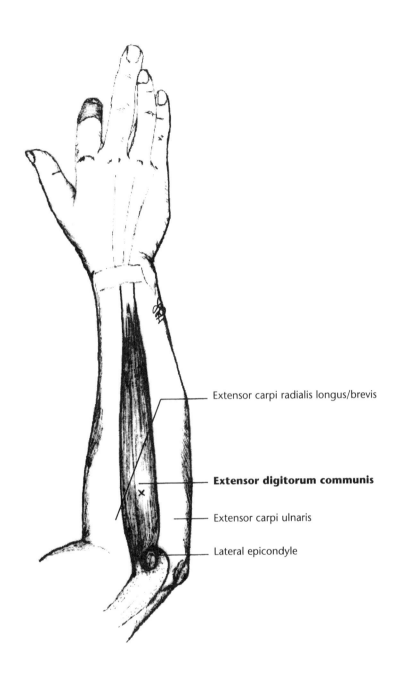

Extensor carpi radialis longus/brevis

Extensor digitorum communis

Extensor carpi ulnaris

Lateral epicondyle

23. Extensor Indicis Proprius

Patient position: Supine with the forearm pronated

Needle insertion: Insert the needle into the distal fourth of the forearm immediately lateral to the radial side of the ulna between the tendons of extensor carpi ulnaris and extensor digitorum. Note that muscle contraction at the distal forearm may be seen or palpable by extending and flexing the index finger.

Activation: Extend the index finger.

Clinical notes: This is the most distally located muscle innervated by the radial nerve and the most distal of the forearm extensor muscles. The muscle can be used in an evaluation of radial nerve conduction. If inserted more proximally, the needle will be in the extensor pollicis longus.

Innervation: C7, C8—posterior cord—radial nerve (posterior interosseous nerve)

Origin: Posterior surface of the ulna below the extensor pollicis longus and the posterior interosseous membrane

Insertion: Extensor expansion of the second finger

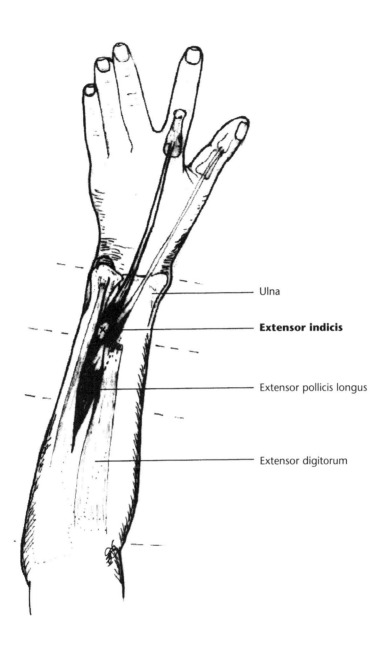

Ulna

Extensor indicis

Extensor pollicis longus

Extensor digitorum

24.   Abductor Pollicis Longus

Patient position: Supine with the forearm pronated and the palm down

Needle insertion: Insert the needle at the junction of the middle and lower third of the dorsal surface of the radius shaft. Before inserting the needle, activation of this muscle (abduction and adduction of the thumb) may be helpful to identify the location of the muscle belly.

Activation: Abduct the thumb or extend the thumb at the metacarpal joint.

Clinical notes: Extensor digitorum partly covers this muscle in the forearm. Origin of the muscle is at about the insertion of the supinator and pronator teres.

Innervation: C7, C8—posterior cord—radial nerve (posterior interosseous nerve)

Origin: Posterior surface of the lower half of the shaft of the ulna below the anconeus, posterior interosseous membrane and the middle third of the posterior radius just distal to supinator

Insertion: Radial (lateral) side of the base of first metacarpal bone

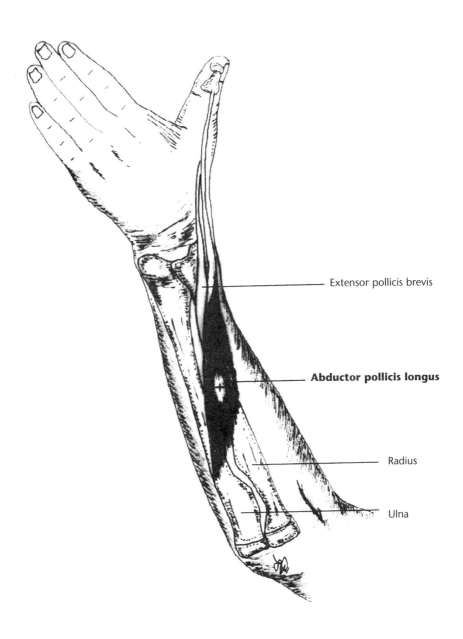

Extensor pollicis brevis

Abductor pollicis longus

Radius

Ulna

25. Extensor Pollicis Longus

Patient position: Supine with the forearm pronated

Needle insertion: Insert the needle at the middle third of the forearm along the radial side of the ulna.

Activation: Extend the thumb (distal phalanx).

Clinical notes: The superficial radial nerve is palpable as it crosses the extensor pollicis longus tendon near the anatomic snuffbox.

Innervation: C7, C8—middle and lower trunk—posterior division—posterior cord—radial nerve (posterior interosseous nerve)

Origin: Posterior surface of the middle third of the ulna shaft and posterior interosseous membrane

Insertion: Dorsal surface of the base of the distal phalanx of the thumb

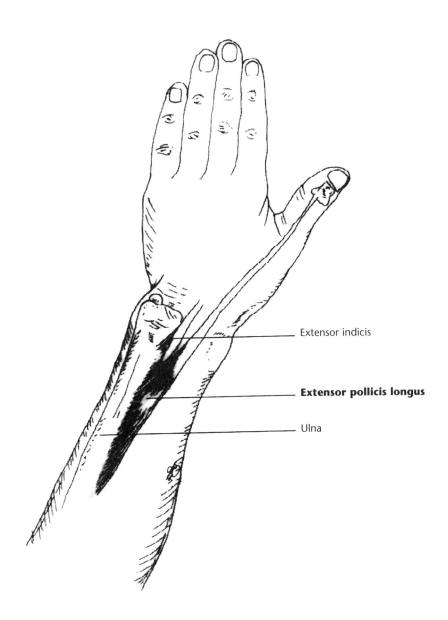

Extensor indicis

Extensor pollicis longus

Ulna

26. Extensor Pollicis Brevis

Patient position: Supine with the forearm pronated

Needle insertion: Insert the needle at the junction of the middle and lower thirds of the posterior surface of the radial shaft, but distal (medial) to the abductor pollicis longus.

Clinical notes: It is a very small and relatively thin layer of muscle. It is closely adherent to the abductor pollicis longus. DeQuervain's tenosynovitis: inflammation of the tendons of the abductor pollicis longus and the extensor pollicis brevis. It is characterized by pain over the radial styloid process and a palpable nodule over the tendons.

Activation: Extension of the proximal phalanx

Innervation: C7, C8—posterior cord—radial nerve (posterior interosseous nerve)

Origin: Posterior surface of the radial shaft below (medial) the abductor pollicis longus and the posterior interosseous membrane

Insertion: Base of the proximal phalanx of the thumb

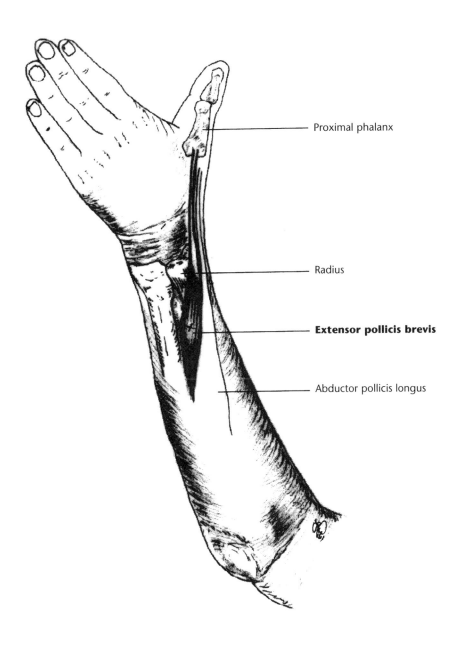

Proximal phalanx

Radius

Extensor pollicis brevis

Abductor pollicis longus

27. Supinator

Patient position: Supine with the forearm pronated

Needle insertion: Insert the needle over the radius between the extensor carpi radialis and the extensor digitorum communis at the upper third of the forearm.

Activation: Supinate the forearm.

Clinical notes: In general, supination is stronger than pronation. When the deep branch of the radial nerve emerges from the supinator, it is referred to as the posterior interosseous nerve. This muscle may or may not be involved in the posterior interosseous syndrome, although it is not involved in supinator syndrome.

Innervation: C5, C6—upper trunk—posterior division—posterior cord—radial nerve (posterior interosseous nerve)

Origin: *Humeral head (superficial head)*—Lateral epicondyle of the humerus, radial collateral ligaments of the elbow joint and annular ligament of the superior radioulnar joint

Ulnar head (deep head)—distal to the radial notch on the posterolateral surface of the ulna, and the supinator fossa and crest of the ulna

Insertion: Humeral head—lateral surface of the radius

Ulnar head—encircles the radius and inserts into the proximal third of the radius

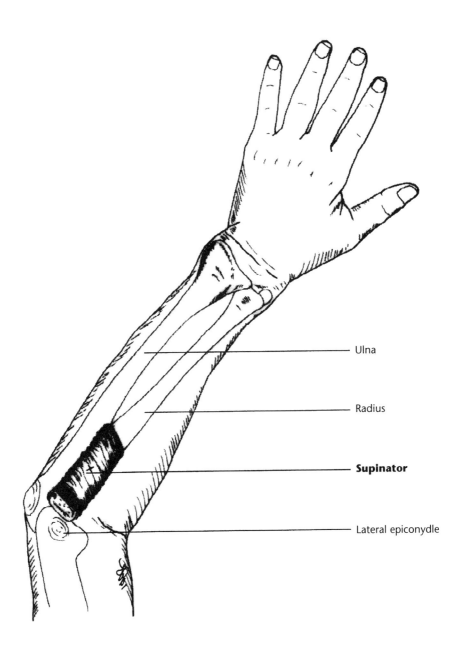

Ulna

Radius

Supinator

Lateral epiconydle

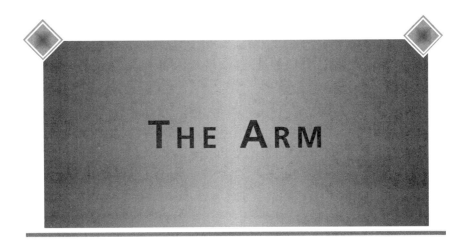

THE ARM

28. Biceps Brachii

Patient position: Supine with the forearm supinated

Needle insertion: Insert the needle just below the midpoint between the shoulder and elbow joint. If the needle is inserted too deeply, it will be in the brachialis.

Activation: Elbow flexion with the forearm fully supinated and with external rotation of the arm. Full activation is not difficult.

Clinical notes: Examined for:

- ♦ C5, C6 radiculopathy
- ♦ Brachial plexus—Upper trunk, lateral cord injury; motor conduction with Erb's point stimulation for either evaluation or brachial plexopathy or isolated pathology
- ♦ Musculocutaneous neuropathy. Watch for volume-conducted response.
- ♦ Myositis/myopathy evaluation

Innervation: C5, C6—upper trunk—lateral cord—musculocutaneous nerve

Origin: *Short head*—coracoid process of the scapula, lateral to the tendon of the coracobrachialis *Long head*—Supraglenoid tubercle of the scapula

Insertion: Radial tuberosity and the lacertus fibrosis (forearm fascia) into the ulnar side of the forearm.

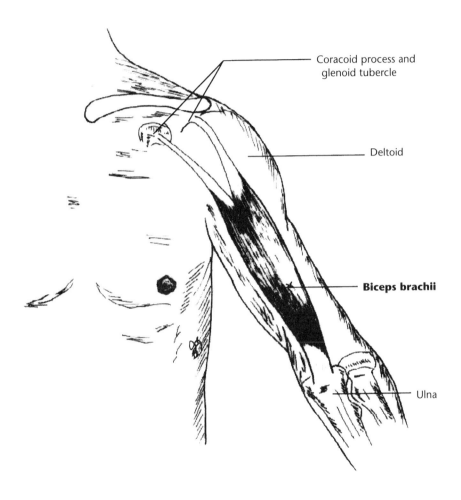

Coracoid process and
glenoid tubercle

Deltoid

Biceps brachii

Ulna

29. Brachialis

Patient position: Supine with the arm at the side of the thorax, elbow slightly flexed, and the forearm pronated

Needle insertion: Note the biceps and brachioradialis at the lower one-third of the arm. At the space between the biceps and brachioradialis at the lower one-third of the arm, the needle is inserted toward the front of the humerus.

Activation: Elbow flexion

Clinical notes: It is found deep to the biceps brachii and is concealed by it in the upper arm. It is the main elbow flexor and is the strongest elbow flexor from the pronated position. Some of the lateral portion of this muscle may be innervated by the radial nerve.

Innervation: C5, C6—upper trunk—lateral cord—musculocutaneous nerve

Origin: Distal half of the anterior humerus, at the insertion of the deltoid, and the intermuscular septum

Insertion: Ulnar tuberosity and the coronoid process of the ulna

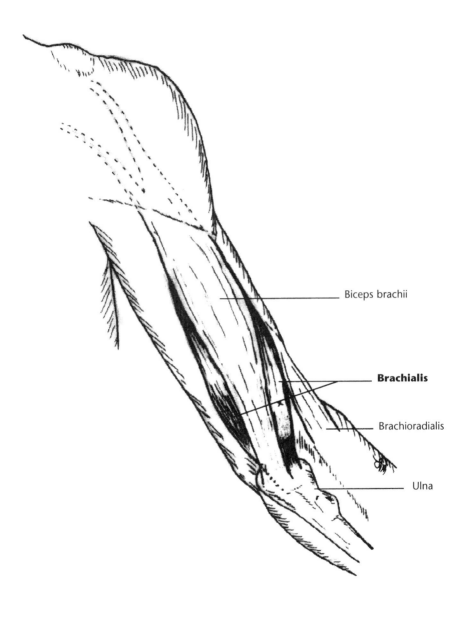

Biceps brachii

Brachialis

Brachioradialis

Ulna

30. Coracobrachialis

Patient position: Supine

Needle insertion: Insert the needle near the junction between the proximal end of the anterior axillary fold (anterior wall) and anterior border of the deltoid muscle. If the needle is inserted too laterally, it will be in the biceps brachii.

Activation: Flex, adduct, and externally rotate the arm with the elbow flexed.

Clinical notes: The musculocutaneous nerve pierces this muscle and may become entrapped. Persistence of the lower head of this muscle is associated with the ligament of Struthers, which attaches from a supratrochlear spur (from the anteromedial aspect of the lower humerus) to the medial epicondyle of the humerus and may entrap the median nerve.

Innervation: C5, C6—upper trunk—lateral cord—musculocutaneous nerve

Origin: Coracoid process of the scapula, in common with the tendon of the short head of biceps

Insertion: Anteromedial surface of the mid-humerus

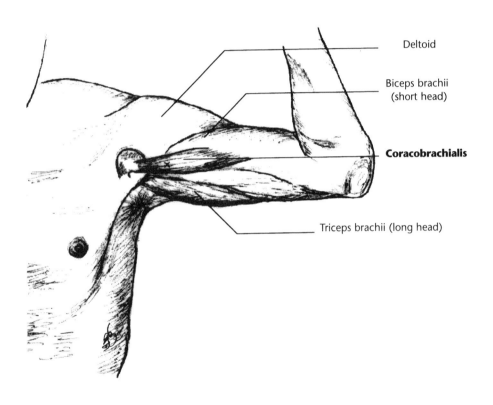

Deltoid

Biceps brachii
(short head)

Coracobrachialis

Triceps brachii (long head)

31. Triceps Brachii

Patient position:　Lateral decubitus, supine or prone

Needle insertion:

1. Long head: Arm abducted at 90 degrees with the elbow extended. At approximately 5 cm distal to the posterior axillary fold and posterior to the posterior deltoid, grasp the muscle belly and insert the needle. The posterior axillary fold is formed by the subscapularis, teres major, and latissimus dorsi.

2. Medial head: Arm internally rotated and the forearm extended. Insert the needle approximately 5 cm straight above the olecranon.

3. Lateral head: Insert the needle just posterior to the deltoid tubercle at the midpoint of the arm.

Activation:　Elbow extension

Clinical notes:　This is the only muscle on the posterior surface of the arm and is the primary elbow extensor. Wrist drop is common resulting from radial nerve compression in the spiral groove. A needle EMG of all three heads and the anconeus is usually normal. Order of recruitment is the medial first, then the lateral, and finally the long head as increased power is needed.

Innervation:　C6, C7, C8—middle and lower trunk— posterior division—radial nerve

Origin:

Long head: Infraglenoid tuberosity of the scapula

Lateral head: Posterior surgical neck of the humerus above the spiral groove

Medial head: Posteromedial half of the humerus below the spiral groove

Insertion:　Proximal end of the olecranon process of the ulna

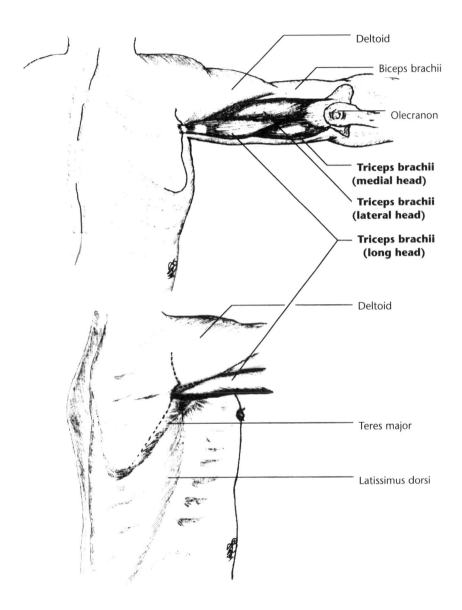

Deltoid

Biceps brachii

Olecranon

Triceps brachii (medial head)

Triceps brachii (lateral head)

Triceps brachii (long head)

Deltoid

Teres major

Latissimus dorsi

32. Anconeus

Patient position: Supine with the elbow flexed and forearm pronated

Needle insertion: Identify the lateral epicondyle of the humerus, olecranon, and proximal ulna. Insert the needle approximately 1 cm distal to the lateral epicondyle and advance it toward the medial border of the ulna.

Activation: Elbow extension

Clinical notes: This muscle is very thin, triangular in shape, and located on the back of the elbow joint. In wrist drop with radial neuropathy in the spiral groove of the humerus, EMG examination of this muscle is usually normal. It is innervated by a branch of the radial nerve that leaves the nerve trunk before entering the spiral groove.

Innervation: C7, C8—posterior cord—radial nerve

Origin: Distal part of the back of the lateral epicondyle of the humerus

Insertion: Lateral surface of the olecranon and the adjacent part of the posterior surface of the ulnar, just above and along the oblique line

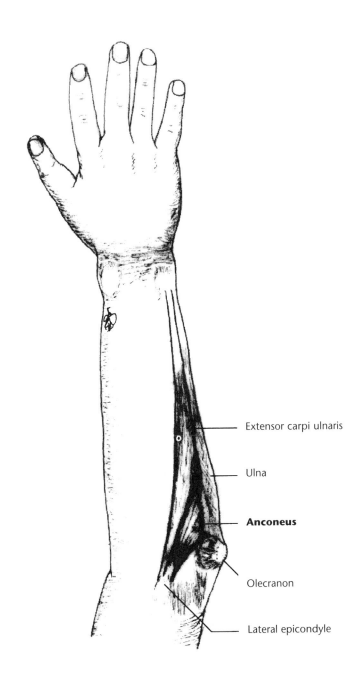

Extensor carpi ulnaris

Ulna

Anconeus

Olecranon

Lateral epicondyle

THE SHOULDER

33. Deltoid

Patient position: Supine, lateral decubitus, or sitting with the arm at the side

Needle insertion: Insert the needle at the midpoint between the humeral tubercle and deltoid tuberosity. Three parts of the muscle (anterior, lateral, and posterior) can be examined with separate needling.

Activation: Flex the arm (anterior deltoid).
Abduct the arm (middle deltoid).
Extend the arm (posterior deltoid).

Clinical notes: Thick, triangular muscle responsible for the round contour of the shoulder. Wasting of this muscle results in a very prominent flattened shoulder. It is the most important arm abductor. The muscle may also show abnormal EMG findings due to repeated previous injections. Activation of the deltoid is greatest between 90 and 180 degrees of elevation. Anterior humeral dislocation and surgical neck fractures may injure the axillary nerve resulting in deltoid paralysis and wasting.

Innervation: C5, C6—Upper trunk—posterior cord—axillary nerve

Origin: Anterior aspect of the lateral third of the clavicle, lateral borders of the acromion, and crest of the scapular spine

Insertion: Deltoid tuberosity of the humerus

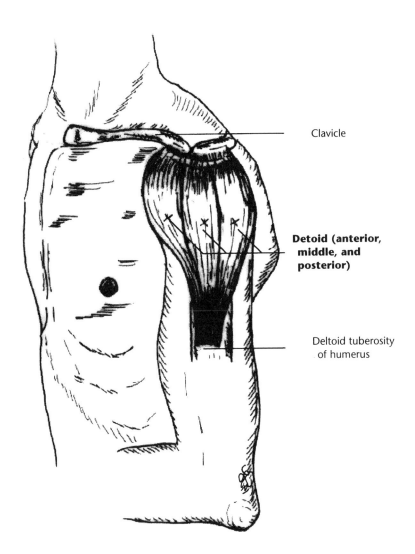

Clavicle

Detoid (anterior, middle, and posterior)

Deltoid tuberosity of humerus

34. Supraspinatus

Patient position:	Lateral decubitus, prone, or sitting
Needle insertion:	The supraspinatus fossa is palpable between the medial half of the spine of the scapula and the upper trapezius. The needle is inserted into the fossa until it reaches the bone, and then is withdrawn slightly. The needle should pass through the trapezius to reach the supraspinatus in the scapular spinous fossa.
Activation:	Abduct the arm at the shoulder.
Clinical notes:	Along with the infraspinatus, subscapularis, and teres minor, it comprises the rotator cuff muscles. Examined for:

♦ Brachial plexopathy—upper trunk lesion
♦ Suprascapular neuropathy
♦ C5 radiculopathy

Innervation:	C5, C6—upper trunk—suprascapular nerve
Origin:	Medial two-thirds of the supraspinous fossa of the scapula
Insertion:	Greater tubercle of the humerus

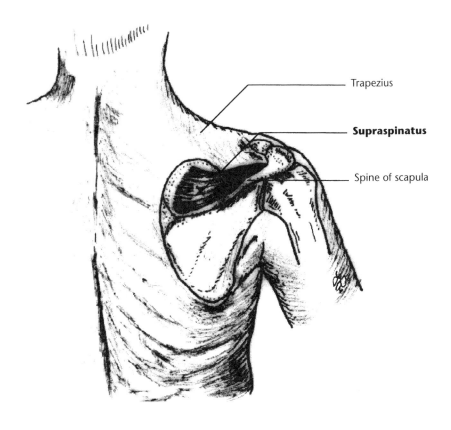

Trapezius

Supraspinatus

Spine of scapula

35. Infraspinatus

Patient position: Lateral decubitus, prone, or sitting

Needle insertion: Note the spine, medial and lateral border of the scapula. Insert the needle approximately 2 to 3 cm below from the scapular spine in the lateral half of the scapula. If the needle is inserted close to the medial border, it must pass through the lower trapezius to reach the infraspinatus.

Activation: Externally rotate the arm with the forearm flexed

Clinical notes: Thick, triangular muscle that occasionally is fused with the teres minor. It is the strongest of the humeral external rotators. Examined for:

♦ C5 radiculopathy
♦ Upper trunk lesion of the brachial plexus
♦ Suprascapular neuropathy

Innervation: C5, C6—upper trunk—suprascapular nerve

Origin: Medial two-thirds of the infraspinous fossa of the scapula

Insertion: Greater tubercle of the humerus

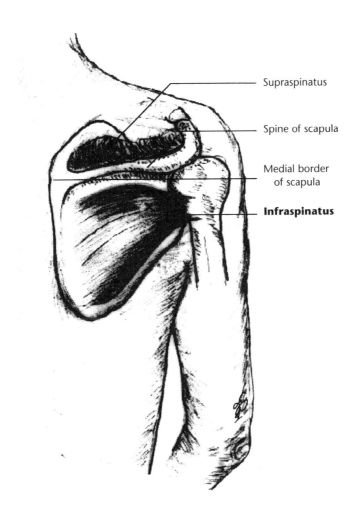

Supraspinatus

Spine of scapula

Medial border
of scapula

Infraspinatus

36. Teres Major

Patient position: Lateral decubitus or prone

Needle insertion: Note the lateral border and lower angle of the scapula, proximal humerus, and posterior axillary fold. Grasp the posterior axillary fold with your thumb and index finger at its lower third and insert the needle in the space between these two fingers and advance it toward the lateral border of the scapula.

Activation: Extend, adduct, and internally rotate the arm. Forearm flexed while moving the hand toward the ipsilateral buttock.

Clinical note: Thick muscle that helps form the posterior axillary fold

Innervation: C5, C6—upper trunk—posterior cord—lower subscapular nerve

Origin: Dorsal inferior angle (lower third of the lateral border) of the scapula

Insertion: Medial lip of the bicipital groove of the humerus, posterior to the tendon of the latissimus dorsi

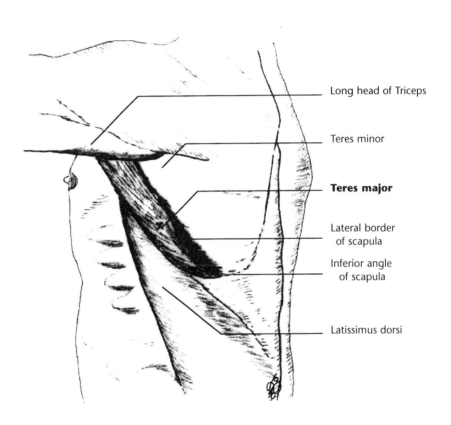

Long head of Triceps

Teres minor

Teres major

Lateral border
of scapula

Inferior angle
of scapula

Latissimus dorsi

37. Teres Minor

Patient position: Lateral decubitus or prone

Needle insertion: Note the lateral border of the scapula and proximal humerus. Insert the needle at the upper third of the scapula, just off its lateral border.

Clinical notes: The muscle is small, short, and narrow, and is attached to the lateral border of the scapula. It is invested by the fascia of the infraspinatus and sometimes is inseparable from the muscle. The long head of the triceps passes under this muscle at the axilla and the teres major passes just lateral to the muscle. The teres minor and infraspinatus are occasionally fused. Technically it is not easy to needle this muscle.

Activation: External rotation of the arm with the forearm flexed

Innervation: C5, C6—upper trunk—posterior cord—axillary nerve

Origin: Upper two-thirds of the dorsal surface of the lateral border of scapula

Insertion: Greater tubercle of humerus, below the insertion of the infraspinatus

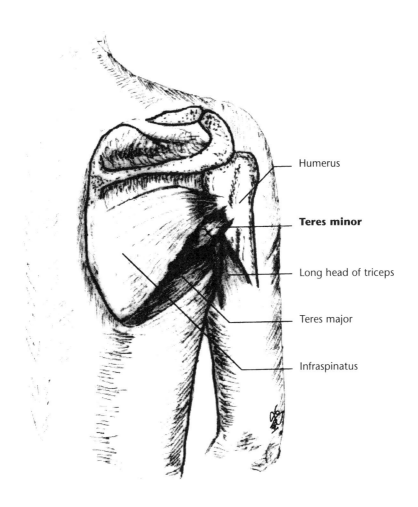

Humerus

Teres minor

Long head of triceps

Teres major

Infraspinatus

38. Rhomboid Major

Patient position: Lateral decubitus or prone

Needle insertion: Identify the lower medial border (just above lower angle) of the scapula and the ribs at the corresponding level of the spinous processes of T2–5. Insert the needle close to the lower medial border of the scapula with care.

Activation: Arm is placed along side of body, elbow flexed, forearm placed behind back. Ask the patient to elevate the medial border and adduct the scapula toward the vertebrae.

Clinical notes: This muscle is located deep to the trapezius. It is believed that the findings in this muscle are comparable with those of corresponding paraspinal muscles because of direct nerve supply of C5. The muscle examination requires great technical experience and care to avoid a pneumothorax.

Innervation: C5 (occasionally from C4)—dorsal scapular nerve

Origin: Thoracic vertebral spinous processes two through five

Insertion: Medial border between the triangular surface at the root of the scapular spine and the inferior angle of the scapula

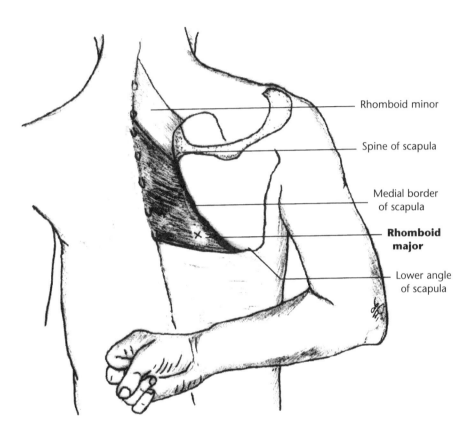

Rhomboid minor

Spine of scapula

Medial border
of scapula

**Rhomboid
major**

Lower angle
of scapula

39. Rhomboid Minor

Patient position:	Prone or side-lying
Needle insertion:	Halfway (closer to the scapula) between the C7 spine and medial end (base) of the spine of the scapula
Activation:	Retract and elevate the scapula.
Clinical notes:	The muscle is deep to the trapezius and is occasionally fused with the rhomboid major. Along with the rhomboid major, the only muscle innervated by a single nerve root.
Innervation:	C5—dorsal scapular nerve—may also have C4
Origin:	Lower part of ligamentum nuchae, and vertebral spinous processes C7 and T1 vertebrae
Insertion:	Medial border at the base (end) of the scapular spine

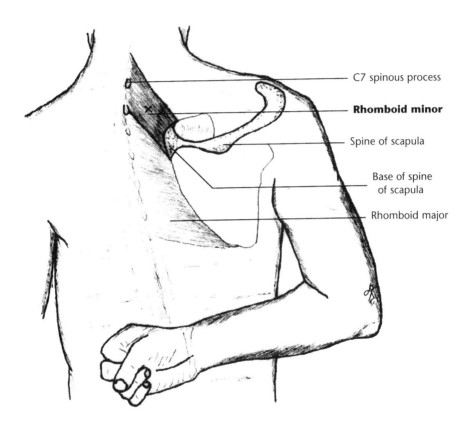

C7 spinous process

Rhomboid minor

Spine of scapula

Base of spine
of scapula

Rhomboid major

40. Levator Scapulae

Patient position:	Side-lying or sitting
Needle insertion:	Turn the head and neck to the opposite side of the muscle being examined and gently raise the same side of the shoulder toward its corresponding ear. You can identify the lateral border of the sternocleidomastoid and the anterior border of the upper trapezius at the superior angle of the posterior superior clavicular fossa. At this area, you can identify the levator scapulae and insert the needle.
Activation:	Ask the patient to elevate his/her shoulder gently toward the ear.
Clinical note:	Straplike muscle that is found deep to the trapezius.
Innervation:	**1.** C3, C4 (cervical plexus) **2.** C5 through the dorsal scapular nerve
Origin:	Transverse processes of the upper four cervical vertebrae
Insertion:	Medial border of the scapula between the superior angle and the medial end (root) of the spine

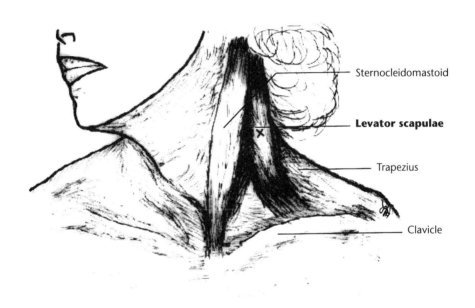

Sternocleidomastoid

Levator scapulae

Trapezius

Clavicle

41 (A). Pectoralis Major—Clavicular Head

Patient position:	Supine
Needle insertion:	With the arm at 90 degree flexion and external rotation, the muscle bulk can be palpated on the anterior aspect to the delto-pectoral groove. Insert the needle into the muscle belly.
Activation:	Adduct, flex, and internally rotate the shoulder (arm).
Clinical notes:	Congenital absence of this muscle has been reported and the surrounding muscles (e.g., deltoid and coracobrachialis) can compensate for the shoulder motion in the absence of the pectoralis major.
Innervation:	C5, C6—upper trunk—lateral cord—lateral pectoral nerve
Origin:	Medial two-thirds of the clavicle
Insertion:	Lateral lip of intertubercular sulcus of the humerus (folds on itself with the clavicular portion on top)

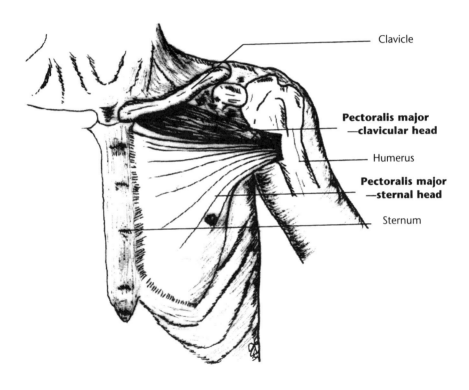

Clavicle

**Pectoralis major
—clavicular head**

Humerus

**Pectoralis major
—sternal head**

Sternum

41 (B). Pectoralis Major—Sternocostal Head

Patient position: Supine

Needle insertion: Grasp the anterior axillary fold by the thumb and index fingers, and insert the needle at the mid-portion of the anterior axillary fold.

Activation: Adduct and internally rotate the arm at shoulder. The palm of hand is placed over the ipsilateral lower chest wall and some pressure is applied to the chest wall to activate the muscle.

Clinical note: Large superficial fan-shaped muscle of the chest wall

Innervation: C7, C8, and T1—middle and lower trunk— medial cord—medial pectoral nerve

Origin: Sternum and upper six costal cartilages

Insertion: Lateral lip of the bicipital groove of the humerus (folds on itself with the clavicular portion on top)

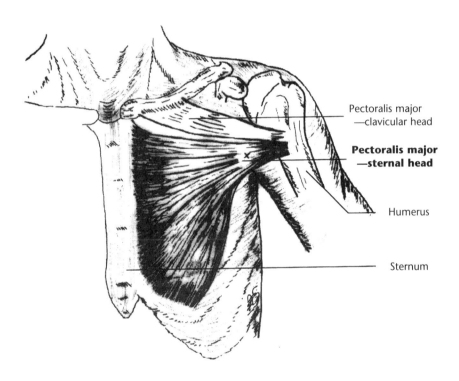

Pectoralis major
—clavicular head

**Pectoralis major
—sternal head**

Humerus

Sternum

42. Pectoralis Minor

Patient position: Supine

Needle insertion: Palpate one of the third, fourth, or fifth ribs in a space between the midclavicular and anterior axillary lines. Insert the needle over one of the ribs while your index and middle fingers are placed over the upper and lower intercostal spaces of that rib, and guide the direction of insertion.

Clinical notes: The majority of this muscle is covered by the pectoralis major. The pectoralis minor is a narrow, flat, triangular muscle that lies in the anterior wall of the axilla. With hyperextension of the arm, the pectoralis minor may entrap the axillary artery and/or the brachial plexus.

Activation: Depression and downward rotation of shoulder

Innervation: C7, C8—medial pectoral nerve

Origin: Midclavicular line of ribs three through five

Insertion: Medial border of the coracoid process of the scapula

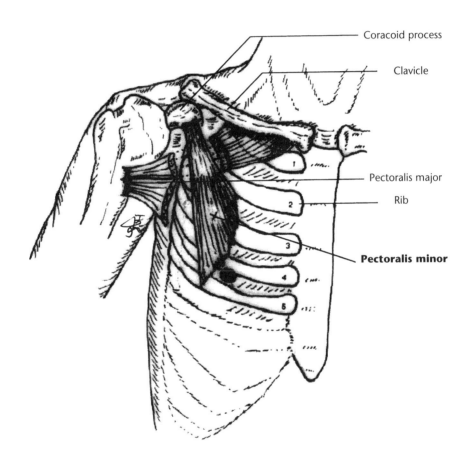

Coracoid process

Clavicle

Pectoralis major

Rib

Pectoralis minor

43. Trapezius

Patient position: Side-lying, sitting, or supine

Needle insertion: Trapezius consists of three parts: upper, middle, and lower. Preferably examine the upper trapezius. At the angle of the neck, grasp the anterior and posterior parts of the muscle belly, and insert the needle and advance it with care.

Activation: Raise the patient's shoulder toward the ear, with his/her upper extremity placed along the side of body.

Clinical notes: Most superficial of the back muscles, and it is thin. In paralysis of the trapezius, one sees lateral winging of the scapula as it is displaced upward and laterally. Examined for:

♦ Accessory neuropathy
♦ Pneumothorax may result with misdirection of the needle.

Innervation: C3, C4 (cervical plexus) but this is generally believed to be sensory, and accessory nerve (C-XI)

Origin (O) and

Insertion (I):

Upper Trapezius:

(O) External occipital tuberance and medial third of the superior nuchal line and spinous process of the seventh cervical vertebra

(I) Lateral one-third of clavicle and acromium

Middle Trapezius:

(O) Spinous processes of the upper thoracic vertebrae, one to five

(I) Superior lip of the scapular spine

Lower Trapezius:

(O) Spinous processes of thoracic vertebrae, six to twelve

(I) Base of the scapular spine

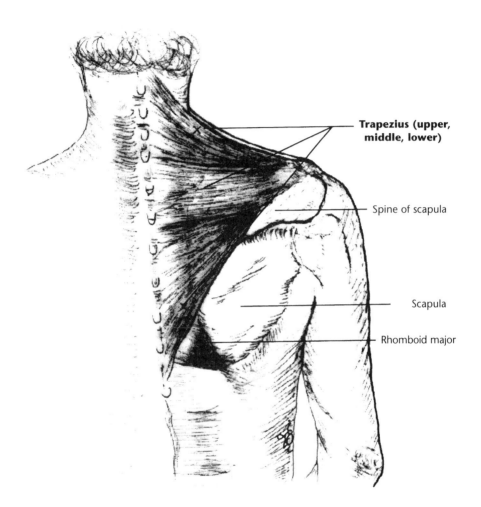

Trapezius (upper, middle, lower)

Spine of scapula

Scapula

Rhomboid major

44. Latissimus Dorsi

Patient position: Lateral decubitus or prone

Needle insertion: With arm abducted, flexed, and externally rotated at the shoulder, this muscle can be identified in the posterior axillary fold. At approximately 5 to 10 cm distal to the axilla, grasp the posterior axillary fold by two fingers and insert the needle more anteriorly (posteriorly; teres major).

Activation: Adduct, extend and internally rotate the humerus against resistance.

Clinical notes: Large, triangular, flat muscle that lies in the lower part of the back. It makes up the largest component of the posterior axillary fold. Along with the pectoralis major, these are the strongest shoulder adductors. It is the most powerful shoulder depressor. Be cautious in order to prevent a pneumothorax. The teres major may be penetrated if the needle is inserted too close to the lateral border of the scapula.

Innervation: C6, C7, C8—posterior cord—thoracodorsal nerve

Origin: Lower six thoracic vertebral spinous processes, all the lumbar vertebral spinous and transverse processes, sacral spinous processes, and the posterior portion of the iliac crest

Insertion: Medial lip of the bicipital groove of the humerus

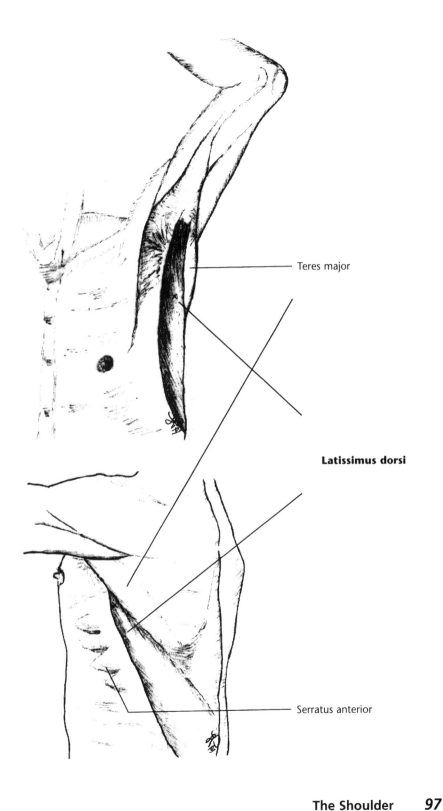

Teres major

Latissimus dorsi

Serratus anterior

45. Serratus Anterior

Patient position: Lateral decubitus or supine with the arm flexed

Needle insertion: Choose one of ribs five through eight near the anterior axillary line, and place two fingers at the adjacent intercostal spaces. Insert the needle into the muscle over the rib at the space between two fingers and advance it with caution, using two fingers to guide the needle.

Activation: Ask the patient to push his/her shoulder forward, drawing the medial border of the scapula anteriorly close to the chest wall. Alternatively, ask the patient to flex his/her arm at 90 degrees with the elbow extended and push forward against the side of a wall, or the examiner's hand.

Clinical notes: Large, curved, quadrilateral-shaped muscle that passes around the thorax and forms the medial wall of the axilla. In paralysis of the serratus anterior, one will see medial winging of the scapula. It is innervated directly by C5, C6, and C7 spinal roots. Its nerve is the first to arise from the spinal roots, and thus it is important to test it in brachial plexus versus root avulsion injuries.

Innervation: C5, C6, and C7 roots—long thoracic nerve

Origin: Outer surface and superior border of ribs 1–8

Insertion: Costal surface of the scapula along the inferior angle and the entire anterior surface of the medial border of the scapula

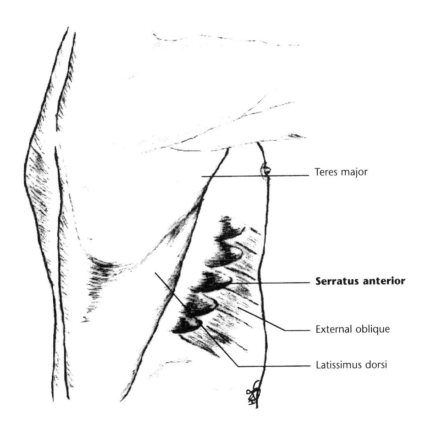

Teres major

Serratus anterior

External oblique

Latissimus dorsi

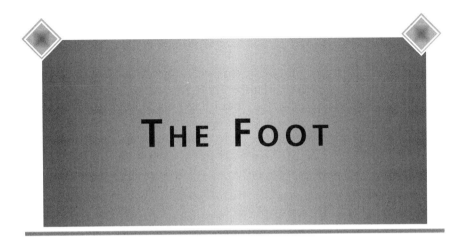

THE FOOT

46. Abductor Hallucis

Patient position: Supine with the foot supinated

Needle insertion: Insert the needle at the medial side of the sole, just inferior to the navicular bone, and advance it toward the lateral border of the foot.

Activation: Abduct and flex the big toe. Ask the patient to curl or fan his/her toes.

Clinical notes: It covers the long tendons that enter the sole of the foot, and covers the origins of the plantar vessels and nerves. Findings of isolated denervation due to repeated local trauma are common. Interpretation of clinical significance of isolated denervation in this muscle is controversial.

Innervation: L5, S1—sciatic nerve—tibial nerve—medial plantar nerve

Origin: Posterior medial tubercle of the calcaneus, the flexor retinaculum, and the plantar aponeurosis

Insertion: Medial side of the flexor plantar surface of the base of the proximal phalanx of the big toe

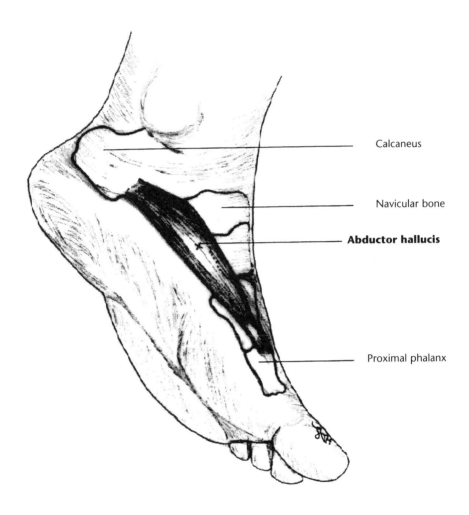

Calcaneus

Navicular bone

Abductor hallucis

Proximal phalanx

47. Flexor Hallucis Brevis

Patient position:	Supine with ankle supinated
Needle insertion:	Insert the needle close to the first metatarsal bone medially, and advance it to the lateral side of foot.
Activation:	Flex the big toe.
Innervation:	L5, S1—tibial nerve—medial plantar nerve
Origin:	Cuneiform bones and divides into two bellies
Insertion:	**Medial belly**—medial side of the base of the proximal phalanx of the big toe and blends with the abductor hallucis
	Lateral belly—lateral side of the base of the proximal phalanx of the big toe and blends with the adductor hallucis

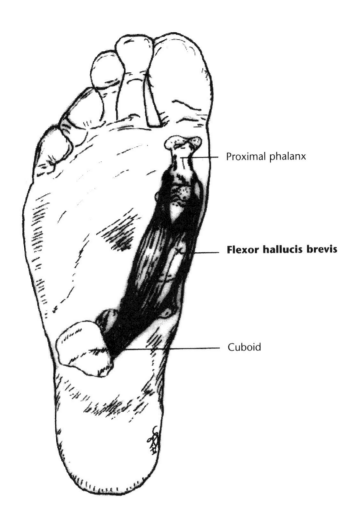

Proximal phalanx

Flexor hallucis brevis

Cuboid

48. Flexor Digitorum Brevis

Patient position: Supine with the foot supinated

Needle insertion: Insert the needle just lateral to the abductor hallucis at the level of the navicular bone and approximately 1 cm off the distal part of the heel pad.

Activation: Flex the middle phalanges.

Clinical notes: This muscle is located deep to the plantar aponeurosis and lateral to the abductor hallucis. This muscle is equivalent to the flexor digitorum superficialis in the upper extremity. The lateral plantar nerves and vessels run deep to this muscle toward the lateral part of the foot.

Innervation: S1, S2—sacral plexus—sciatic nerve—tibial nerve—medial plantar nerve

Origin: Medial tubercle of the calcaneus

Insertion: Sides of the base of the middle phalanx of the lateral four digits (2, 3, 4, 5)

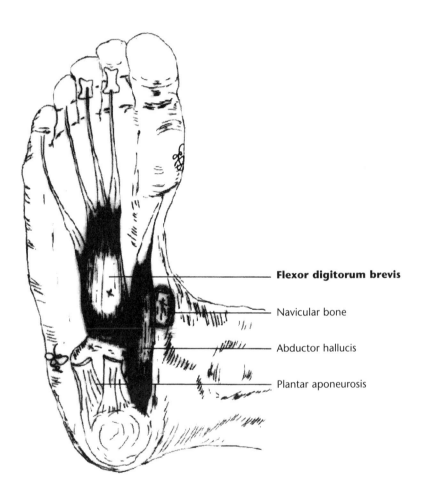

Flexor digitorum brevis

Navicular bone

Abductor hallucis

Plantar aponeurosis

49. Abductor Digiti Minimi

Patient position: Side-lying, or supine with the foot pronated

Needle insertion: Just inferior to the lateral border of the cuneiform bone of the foot

Activation: Ask the subject to flex and fan his/her lateral toes. Also ask the patient to make a cup of his/her foot.

Innervation: S1, S2—sciatic nerve—tibial nerve—lateral plantar nerve

Origin: Lateral tubercle of the calcaneus and the plantar aponeurosis

Insertion: Lateral side of the base of the proximal phalanx of the fifth toe

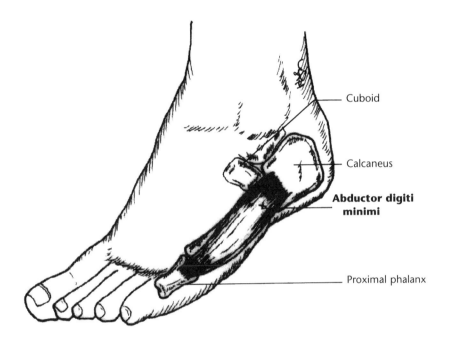

Cuboid

Calcaneus

Abductor digiti minimi

Proximal phalanx

50. First Dorsal Interosseous (Foot)

Patient position: Supine

Needle insertion: Mid-portion of the first web space (space between first and second metatarsal bones)

Activation: Abduct the toes (fan toes out).

Clinical note: The line for reference with respect to abduction or adduction in the foot is the second toe.

Innervation: S1, S2—sciatic nerve—tibial nerve—lateral plantar nerve

Origin: Adjacent sides of the first and second metatarsal bones

Insertion: Medial side of the base of the proximal phalanx of the second toe

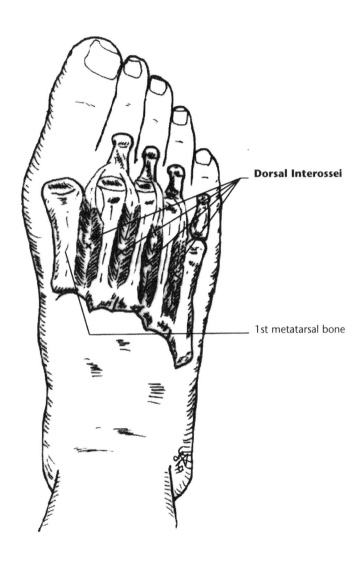

Dorsal Interossei

1st metatarsal bone

51. Extensor Digitorum Brevis

Patient position:	Supine
Needle insertion:	Insert the needle at the proximal one-third of the top of the foot between the tip of the lateral malleolus and the third or fourth toe.
Activation:	Extend the phalanges of the second, third, and fourth toes.
Innervation:	L5, S1—sciatic nerve—common peroneal nerve—deep peroneal nerve
Clinical notes:	Superficial, very thin muscle. Insert the needle at a sharp angle (20 to 30 degrees) to the skin. Denervation limited to this muscle due to repeated trauma is common. In approximately 28% of cases, the lateral portion of this muscle is innervated by the accessory peroneal nerve, which is a branch of the superficial peroneal nerve.
Origin:	Superolateral surface of the calcaneus, extensor retinaculum, and lateral talocalcaneal ligament
Insertion:	Lateral sides of the tendon of the extensor digitorum longus of the second, third, and fourth toes. Also into the dorsal surface of the base of the proximal phalanx of the great toe.

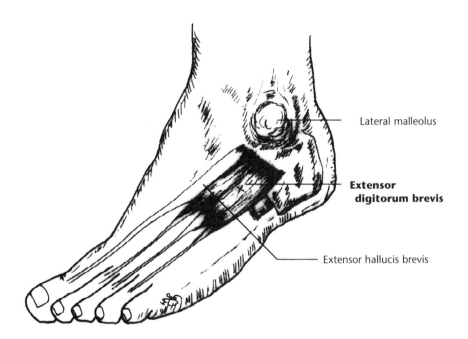

Lateral malleolus

Extensor digitorum brevis

Extensor hallucis brevis

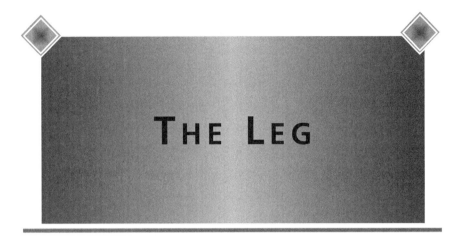

THE LEG

52. Tibialis Anterior

Patient position: Supine

Needle insertion: Insert the needle approximately 1.5 cm lateral to the tibial crest and at the junction of the upper and middle third of the leg.

Activation: Dorsiflex the ankle and invert the foot.

Clinical notes: Tibialis anterior tendon is the most prominent and most medial of the dorsal three tendons. Examined for:

- ♦ Foot drop due to either common peroneal neuropathy or L5 radiculopathy
- ♦ Unspecified lower extremity pain
- ♦ Repetitive stimulation for myasthenic syndrome (stimulate the common peroneal nerve at the fibular head area).

Innervation: L4, L5, (S1)—peroneal portion of sciatic nerve—common peroneal nerve—deep peroneal nerve

Origin: Lateral condyle of tibia, upper two-thirds of the lateral tibial surface and anterior interosseous membrane

Insertion: Dorsal medial side of the first (medial) cuneiform and base of first metatarsal bone

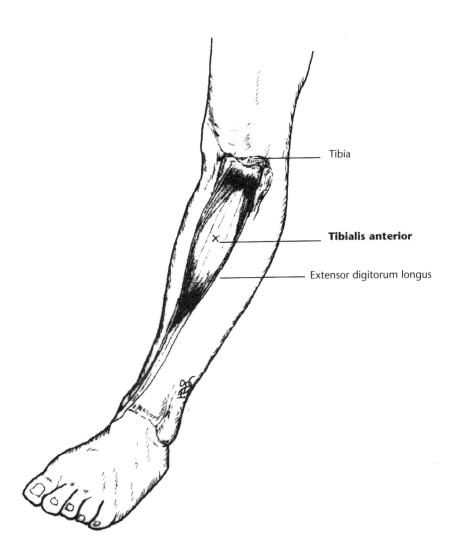

Tibia

Tibialis anterior

Extensor digitorum longus

53. Extensor Digitorum Longus

Patient position: Supine or side-lying

Needle insertion: At the middle third of the leg, a needle is inserted midway between the anterior border of the tibia and lateral border of the fibula

Activation: Extend the toes and dorsiflex the ankle.

Clinical notes: Muscle belly is the most lateral of the anterior compartment muscles. Its tendons are joined by the tendons of the extensor digitorum brevis. If a needle is inserted too medially, it will be in the tibialis anterior; too deeply, in the extensor hallucis longus.

Innervation: L5 and S1—deep peroneal nerve

Origin: Anterolateral tibial condyle, anterior proximal three-fourths of the fibula, and the adjacent anterior interosseous membrane

Insertion: Middle and distal phalanges of the lateral four digits, forming a membranous expansion over the dorsum of each respective metatarsophalangeal joint where it fuses with the capsule. Near the proximal interphalangeal joint, the expansion divides into three slips. The central part of the aponeurosis continues distally to the dorsal base of the middle phalanx. Collateral slips continue to the base of the distal phalanx.

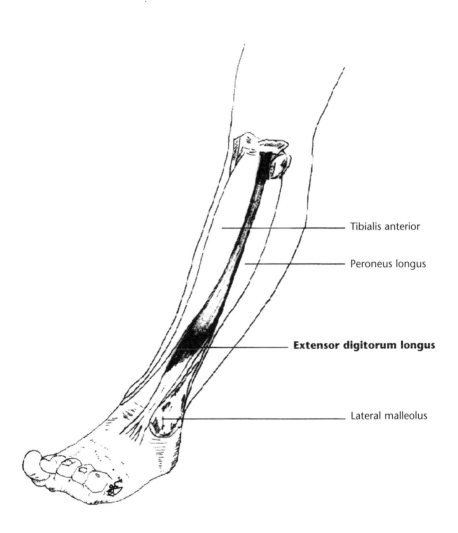

Tibialis anterior

Peroneus longus

Extensor digitorum longus

Lateral malleolus

54. Extensor Hallucis Longus

Patient position: Supine or side-lying

Needle insertion: At the junction between the middle and lower third of the tibia, and at the space between the tendons of the tibialis anterior and extensor digitorum longus. The extensor digitorum longus tendon may be pushed laterally and the needle advanced toward the anterior surface of the fibula, with extension of the big toe and ankle dorsiflexion.

Activation: Extend the big toe.

Clinical notes: This muscle is commonly tested to assess L5 radiculopathy and foot drop. The muscle lies between the tibialis anterior and extensor digitorum longus, somewhat above the ankle.

Innervation: L5, S1—peroneal part of sciatic nerve— common peroneal nerve—deep peroneal nerve

Origin: Middle third of anterior surface of fibula and the adjacent anterior interosseous membrane

Insertion: Dorsum of the base of the distal phalanx of the big toe

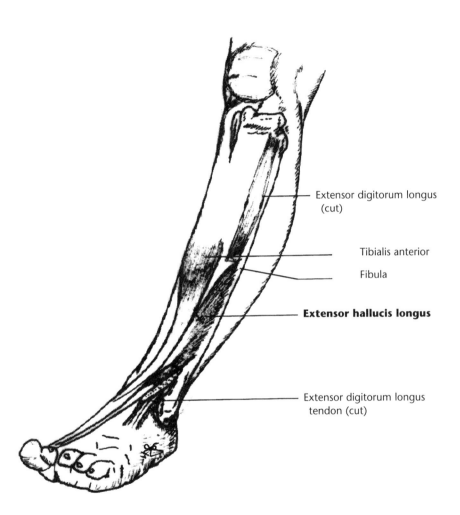

Extensor digitorum longus (cut)

Tibialis anterior

Fibula

Extensor hallucis longus

Extensor digitorum longus tendon (cut)

55. Peroneus Tertius

Patient position: Side-lying

Needle insertion: Insert the needle at the anteromedial border of the fibula between the extensor digitorum longus and the peroneus brevis at the junction of the middle and lower third of the leg.

Activation: Dorsiflex the ankle and evert the foot.

Clinical note: Shares a common origin with the extensor digitorum longus. It is very variable in size and may be congenitally absent.

Innervation: L5, S1—deep peroneal nerve

Origin: Lower third of the anterior fibula with the extensor digitorum longus and the anterior aspect of the interosseous membrane

Insertion: Medial part of the dorsal aspect of the base of the fifth metatarsal bone

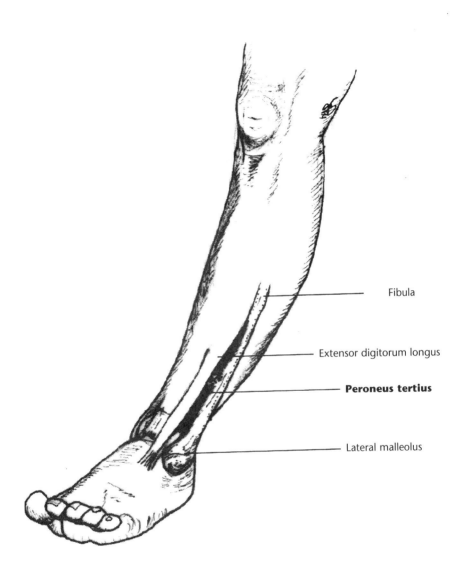

Fibula

Extensor digitorum longus

Peroneus tertius

Lateral malleolus

56. Peroneus Longus

Patient position:	Side-lying or supine
Needle insertion:	At approximately 5 to 10 cm inferior from the fibula neck, place two fingers (thumb and index) over the anterior and lateral surfaces of the fibula, insert the needle into the space between the two fingers, and advance it toward the fibula.
Activation:	Plantar-flexion of the ankle and eversion of the foot
Clinical notes:	In common peroneal neuropathy at the fibular head, this muscle is often less involved than the tibialis anterior. This muscle covers the lateral surface of the fibula, and along with the peroneus brevis forms the lateral compartment of the calf. If the needle is inserted too medially, it will be in the extensor digitorum longus; too posteriorly, the soleus or gastrocnemius.
Innervation:	L5 and S1—peroneal portion of sciatic nerve— common peroneal nerve—superficial peroneal nerve
Origin:	Head and proximal two-thirds of the lateral surface of the fibula
Insertion:	Lateral aspect of the base of the first metatarsal bone and medial (first) cuneiform

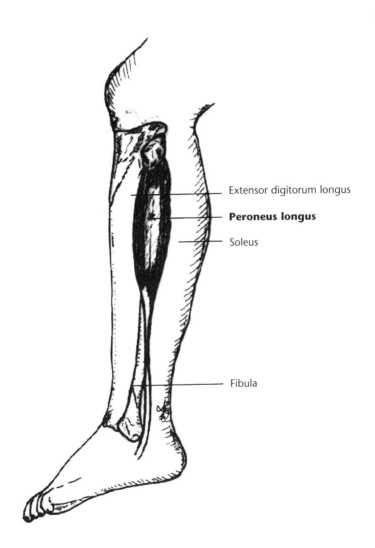

Extensor digitorum longus

Peroneus longus

Soleus

Fibula

57. Peroneus Brevis

Patient position: Supine or side-lying

Needle insertion: At the anterolateral border of the fibula, the needle is inserted at the junction of the middle and lower thirds of the fibula. The proximal part of this muscle lies deep to the peroneus longus.

Clinical note: It lies deep to the peroneus longus.

Activation: Plantar flexion of the ankle and eversion of the foot

Innervation: L5 and S1—superficial peroneal nerve

Origin: Distal two-thirds of the lateral surface of the fibula and the intermuscular fascia

Insertion: Dorsal lateral aspect of the base of the fifth metatarsal bone

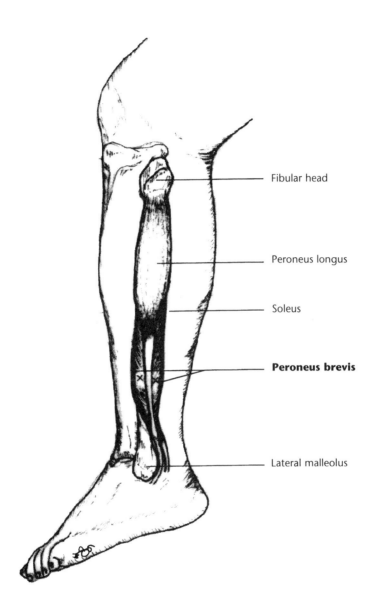

Fibular head

Peroneus longus

Soleus

Peroneus brevis

Lateral malleolus

58. Gastrocnemius

Patient position: Supine, side-lying, or prone

Needle insertion: This muscle has two heads: the medial and lateral. The medial and lateral heads are divided approximately by a line drawn between the midpoint of the popliteal crease and the Achilles tendon at the ankle. Both heads are superficial and easily recognized. The needle is inserted at the center of muscle belly in the head of each side.

Activation: Plantar flexion of the ankle with the knee extended

Clinical notes: The gastrocnemius is the most superficial muscle of the calf. This muscle covers most of the soleus muscle. Together with the soleus muscle, it is called the triceps surae. The medial head is easily tested even in supine position and is more frequently examined than the lateral head. If the needle is inserted too deeply, it could be in any muscle depending on the direction and depth: soleus, flexor digitorum longus, flexor hallucis longus, or tibialis posterior. The tibial nerve passes deep to the muscle.

Innervation: S1, S2—sciatic nerve (tibial portion)—tibial nerve

Origin: **Lateral head:** Proximal aspect of the lateral femoral condyle

Medial head: Popliteal surface of the femur proximal to the medial epicondyle

Insertion: Achilles tendon to the calcaneus—(common tendon with soleus)

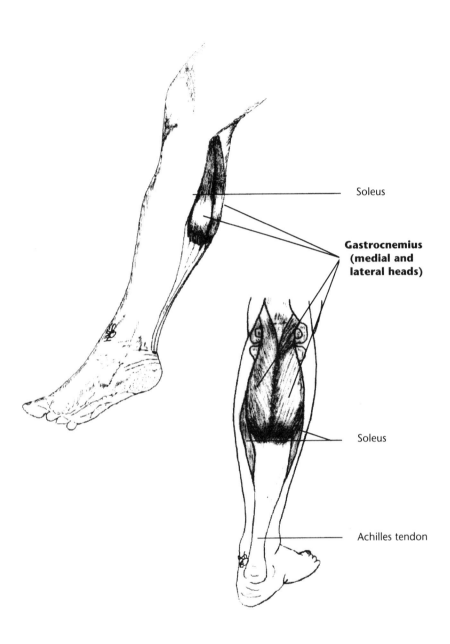

Soleus

**Gastrocnemius
(medial and
lateral heads)**

Soleus

Achilles tendon

The Leg *129*

59. Soleus

Patient position:	Side-lying or prone
Needle insertion:	From the medial side of the calf in a side-lying position, insert the needle just below and at the anterior aspect of the lower margin of the gastrocnemius muscle belly.
Activation:	Plantar flexion of the ankle
Clinical notes:	Broad, flat muscle located deep to the gastrocnemius.
	Medial approach: If the needle is inserted too medially or too deeply, it could be in either the flexor digitorum longus or tibialis posterior.
	Lateral approach: If inserted too deeply, it will be in the flexor hallucis longus.
Innervation:	S1, S2—sciatic nerve—tibial nerve
Origin:	1. Fibular head—proximal posterior upper third of the fibula
	2. Tibial head—proximal third of the posterior tibia
Insertion:	Achilles tendon to the calcaneus—(common tendon with gastrocnemius)

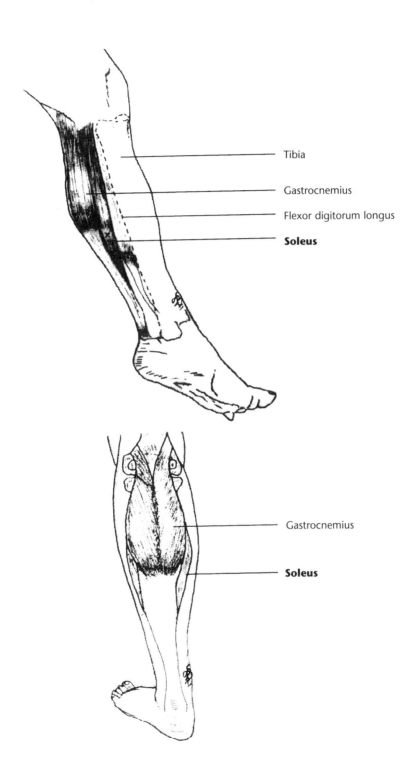

Tibia

Gastrocnemius

Flexor digitorum longus

Soleus

Gastrocnemius

Soleus

60. Flexor Digitorum Longus

Patient position:	Supine
Needle insertion:	At the midway point of the calf, insert the needle just posterior and off the medial border of the tibia. Advance it toward the posterior surface of the tibia.
Activation:	Flex the lateral four toes with plantar flexion of the ankle and inversion of the foot.
Clinical notes:	This muscle is the most medial of the three posterior calf muscles. Its tendons give rise to the lumbrical muscles. Its action is similar to the flexor digitorum profundus of the forearm. Examined for:

♦ L5 radiculopathy or unspecified lower extremity pain. The tibialis posterior and this muscle have the same innervation: L5, S1, and tibial nerve.

♦ Sciatic or tibial neuropathy

Innervation:	L5, S1—sciatic nerve—tibial nerve
Origin:	Middle third of posterior surface of the tibia
Insertion:	Four tendons to the plantar surfaces of the base of the terminal phalanx of digits two through five

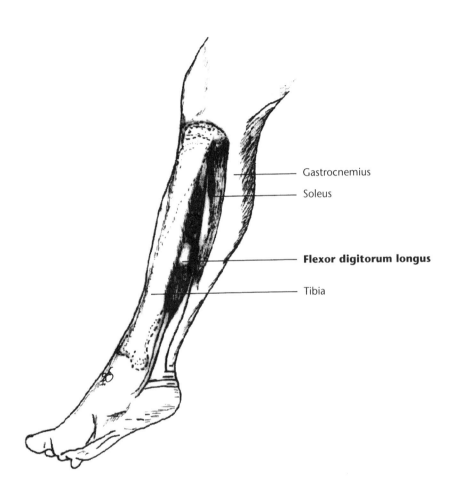

Gastrocnemius

Soleus

Flexor digitorum longus

Tibia

61. Tibialis Posterior

Patient position: Supine

Needle insertion: Insert the needle at the midpoint between the tibia and fibula at the middle third of the leg anteriorly and advance it through either the tibialis anterior or the extensor digitorum longus posteriorly toward the interosseous membrane that is connecting the tibia and the fibula. After passing the interosseous membrane, the needle may reach the tibialis posterior. It requires a long needle, approximately the same length as the distance between the anterior and medial borders of tibia. The authors believe that this approach is more accurate and perhaps safer, as it may avoid penetrating the large neurovascular structures that are located posteriorly to the tibialis posterior.

(*Reference:* Lee HJ, Bach JR, DeLisa JA: *Am J Phys Med Rehabil* 69: 126–127, 1990)

Activation: Plantar flexion of the ankle and inversion of the foot

Clinical notes: The tibialis posterior is the deepest muscle of the posterior compartment group of the calf muscle. Posteriorly, there are neurovascular structures, soleus, and gastrocnemius; medially, the flexor digitorum longus; laterally, the flexor hallucis longus; anteriorly, the interosseous membrane, part of tibialis anterior, extensor digitorum longus, tibia, and fibula. It is an important muscle to assess L5 radiculopathy. With one needle stick, you may check two different muscles (tibialis anterior and posterior), which are innervated by the same L5 root but are innervated by two different peripheral nerves (deep peroneal nerve and tibial nerve).

Innervation: L5 and S1—tibial nerve.

Origin: Lateral aspect of the posterior tibia, proximal two-thirds of the medial posterior fibula, posterior surface of the interosseous membrane, and the intermuscular septum

Insertion: Navicular tuberosity, sustentaculum tali, and the three cuneiforms, cuboid, and plantar surface of bases of second, third, and fourth metatarsals

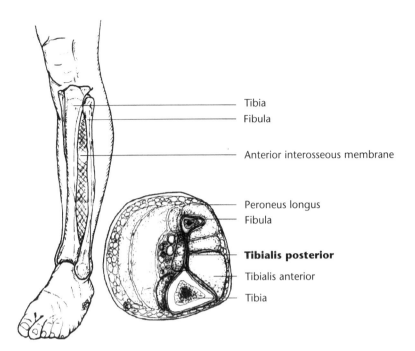

Tibia
Fibula

Anterior interosseous membrane

Peroneus longus
Fibula

Tibialis posterior

Tibialis anterior

Tibia

(Anterior view at the middle of the leg)

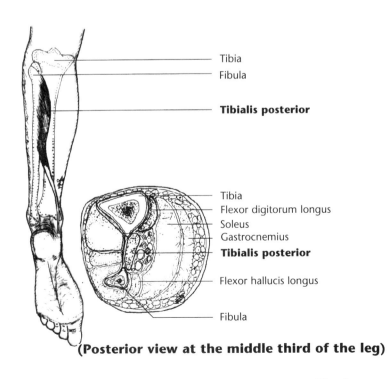

Tibia
Fibula

Tibialis posterior

Tibia
Flexor digitorum longus
Soleus
Gastrocnemius
Tibialis posterior

Flexor hallucis longus

Fibula

(Posterior view at the middle third of the leg)

The Leg   135

62. Flexor Hallucis Longus

Patient position: Side-lying on the opposite side or prone

Needle insertion: Insert the needle close to the posterior surface of the fibula at the mid-half point of the calf laterally.

Activation: Flex the big toe with plantar flexion of the ankle.

Clinical notes: It is the most laterally located of the deep calf muscle group and is the largest of the three deep muscles. It is important in maintaining the medial arch of the foot.

Innervation: S2, S3—tibial nerve

Origin: Distal two-thirds of the posterior surface of the fibula and adjacent interosseous membrane

Insertion: Plantar surface of the base of the distal phalanx of the big toe

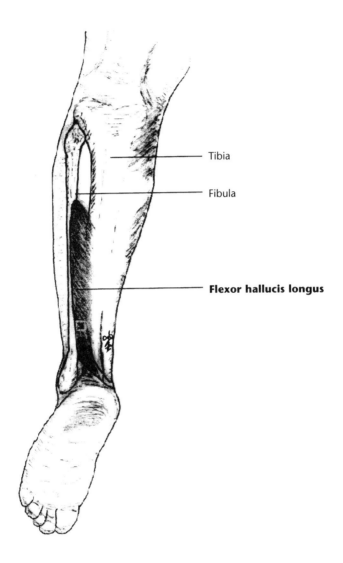

Tibia

Fibula

Flexor hallucis longus

THE ANTERIOR
THIGH

63. Iliopsoas

Patient position: Supine with the hip slightly flexed and the knee in a comfortable position

Needle insertion: Note the femoral artery, anterior superior iliac spine (ASIS), and inguinal ligament. Insert the needle midway between the femoral artery (recognized by palpation of pulse) and ASIS, but just below the inguinal ligament.

Activation: Flex, adduct, and externally rotate the thigh.

Clinical notes: The iliacus is a large, fan-shaped muscle that lies along the lateral side of the psoas major. The psoas major is a long fusiform-shaped muscle. The iliopsoas is the most powerful flexor of the thigh. The lumbar plexus is located within this muscle and the femoral artery descends through the psoas major, then runs between it and the iliacus. If the needle is inserted too laterally, it will be in the sartorius.

Innervation: The iliacus is the most proximal muscle innervated by the femoral nerve (L2, L3), whereas the psoas major is innervated by ventral rami of the first, second, and third lumbar spinal nerves.

Origin: Psoas major from the anterolateral aspect of the bodies and transverse processes of the 12th thoracic and all the lumbar vertebrae and intervertebral disc; Iliacus from the superior aspect of the iliac fossa

Insertion: Lesser trochanter of the femur

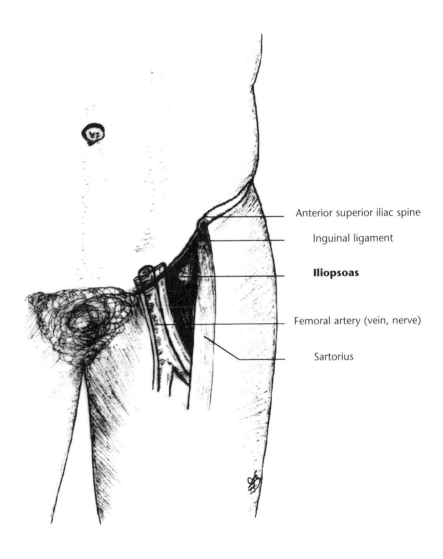

Anterior superior iliac spine

Inguinal ligament

Iliopsoas

Femoral artery (vein, nerve)

Sartorius

64. Pectineus

Patient position: Supine

Needle insertion: Palpate the femoral artery pulse in the inguinal area and insert the needle approximately 1 cm medial to the artery and below the inguinal fossa. If inserted too deeply, it will be in the obturator externus; too medially, in either the gracilis or adductor longus.

Activation: Ask the patient to flex and adduct the hip.

Clinical notes: Flat, quadrilateral-shaped muscle occasionally innervated by the obturator or accessory obturator nerve

Innervation: L2, L3—femoral nerve

Origin: Pectineal line of the pubis

Insertion: Pectoral line of the femur near the medial lip of the upper linea aspera and just below the lesser trochanter of the femur

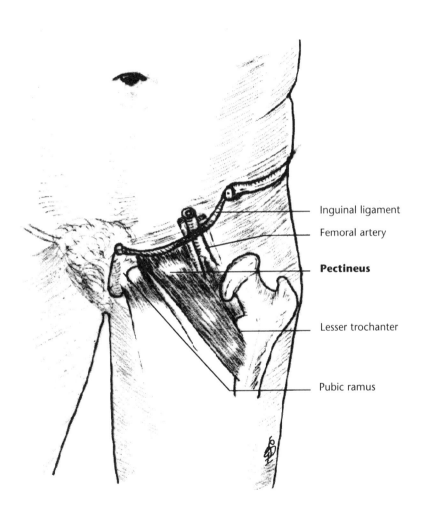

Inguinal ligament

Femoral artery

Pectineus

Lesser trochanter

Pubic ramus

65. Rectus Femoris

Patient position: Supine with the knee extended

Needle insertion: Insert the needle at the middle third of the femur anteriorly and halfway between the medial and lateral border of the thigh.

Activation: Flex the hip with the knee extended.

Clinical notes: Flat, spindle-shaped muscle. It is the only "quadriceps" muscle that crosses two joints. It is located at the middle aspect of the anterior thigh. If the needle is inserted too deeply, it will be in the vastus intermedius.

Innervation: L2, L3, L4—femoral nerve

Origin: Anterior inferior iliac spine, upper lip of the acetabulum, and the fibrous capsule of the hip joint

Insertion: Base of the patella and into the tibial tuberosity by the patellar ligament

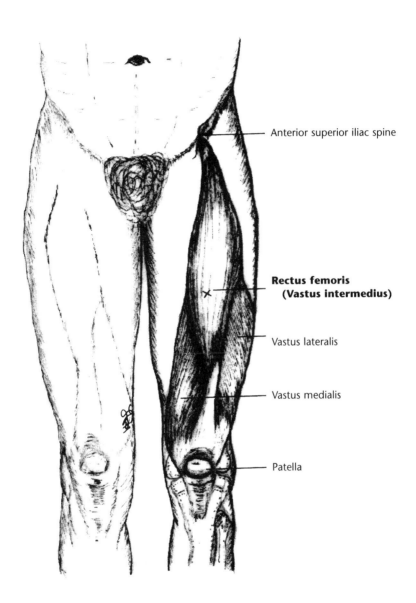

Anterior superior iliac spine

Rectus femoris (Vastus intermedius)

Vastus lateralis

Vastus medialis

Patella

66. Vastus Medialis

Patient position: Supine with the knee extended

Needle insertion: Insert the needle approximately 5 to 10 cm straight above the medial border of the patella.

Activation: Extend the knee. Ask the patient to push the kneecap down on the examination table.

Clinical notes: Located on the medial aspect of the anterior thigh. Its fibers run downward and forward. This muscle is often used for femoral nerve conduction.

Innervation: L2, L3, L4—femoral nerve

Origin: Medial lip of the linea aspera of the femur; intertrochanteric line of the femur and the medial intermuscular septum.

Insertion: Medial aspect of the patella and into the tibial tuberosity by the patellar ligament. Some horizontal fibers insert into the lower part of the medial border of the patella.

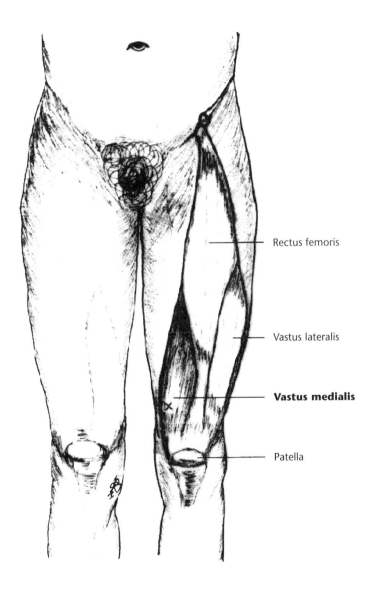

Rectus femoris

Vastus lateralis

Vastus medialis

Patella

67. Vastus Lateralis

Patient position: Supine

Needle insertion: Insert the needle at the junction of the middle and lower third of the thigh straight above the lateral border of the patella.

Activation: Extend the knee.

Clinical notes: It is a broad, thick muscle and is the largest of the quadriceps group. It is located on the lateral aspect of the anterior thigh.

Innervation: L2, L3, L4—femoral nerve

Origin: Upper one-half of the lateral lip of the linea aspera of the femur, greater trochanter of the femur, and intertrochanteric line of the femur

Insertion: Lateral aspect of the patella and into the tibial tuberosity by the patellar ligament

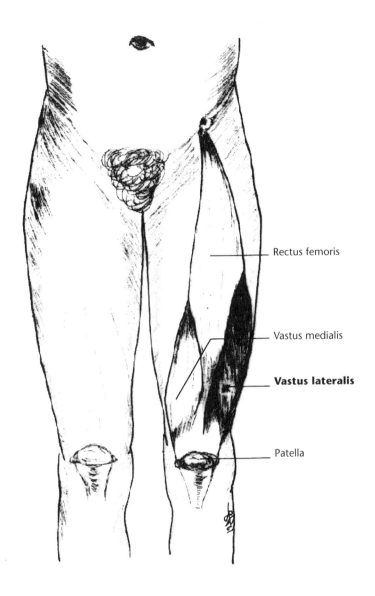

Rectus femoris

Vastus medialis

Vastus lateralis

Patella

68. Sartorius

Patient position: Supine with the hip flexed, abducted, and externally rotated, and the knee flexed. Place the testing leg over the opposite leg.

Needle insertion: Note the anterior superior iliac spine (ASIS) and medial condyle of the femur. Insert the needle approximately 5 to 10 cm distal to the ASIS in a line drawn between the ASIS and the medial condyle.

Activation: Flex, externally rotate, and abduct the hip, flex the knee.

Clinical notes: It is the longest muscle in the body and has the longest fibers. It descends obliquely across the front and medial sides of the thigh. The common insertion of the sartorius, gracilis, and semitendinosus forms the pes anserinus. If the needle is inserted too medially, it will be in the iliopsoas: too deeply, in the rectus femoris: too laterally, in the tensor fascia lata.

Innervation: L2, L3—femoral nerve

Origin: Anterior superior iliac spine

Insertion: Upper medial surface of the tibia, anterior to the insertion of the gracilis and the semitendinosus

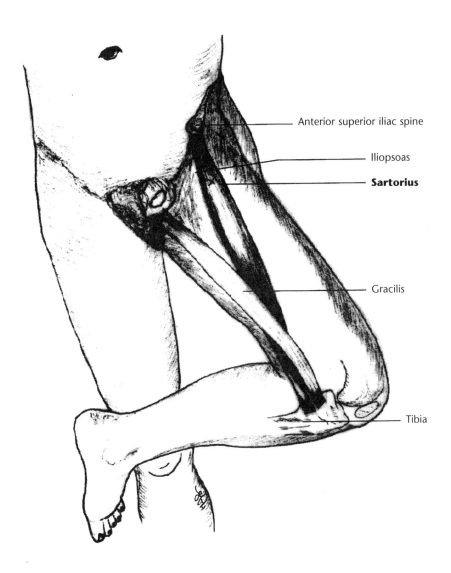

Anterior superior iliac spine

Iliopsoas

Sartorius

Gracilis

Tibia

69. Tensor Fascia Lata

Patient position: Side-lying or supine

Needle insertion: Insert the needle at approximately 3 to 4 cm posterior along the line of iliac crest from the anterior superior iliac spine (ASIS), and approximately 5 to 10 cm inferior directly from iliac crest toward the front of the greater trochanter of the femur.

Activation: Abduct and internally rotate the hip or abduct the hip with the knee extended.

Clinical notes: It is a thin muscle at its origin that becomes thicker at its insertion into the iliotibial tract. The iliotibial band also receives fibers from the gluteus maximus. It is triangular in shape and is enclosed between the two layers of the fascia lata. Examined for:

♦ L5 radiculopathy.

♦ Unspecified leg pain

♦ Superior gluteal neuropathy

Innervation: L4, L5, S1—superior gluteal nerve

Origin: Anterior portion of the outer lip of the iliac crest and the anterior superior iliac spine

Insertion: Iliotibial tract to the lateral condyle of the tibia

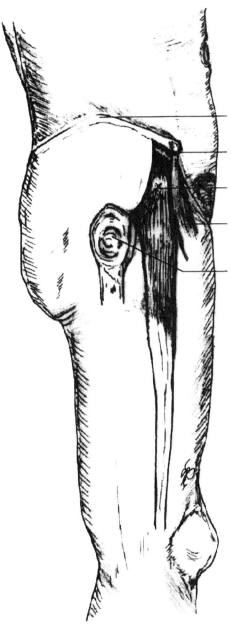

Iliac crest

Anterior superior iliac spine

Tensor fascia lata

Sartorius

Greater trochanter

The Anterior Thigh   153

70. Adductor Longus

Patient position: Supine with the hip abducted, slightly flexed, and the knee flexed. The testing leg is placed over the opposite leg.

Needle insertion: Insert the needle at the junction of the upper and middle third of the medial thigh in a space between the sartorius and gracilis muscle.

Activation: Adduct the thigh from the above patient position.

Clinical note: It is triangular in shape and is the most superficial muscle of the adductor group.

Innervation: L2, L3, L4—obturator nerve (anterior division)

Origin: Pubic tubercle

Insertion: Medial lip of the lower two-thirds of the linea aspera of the femur

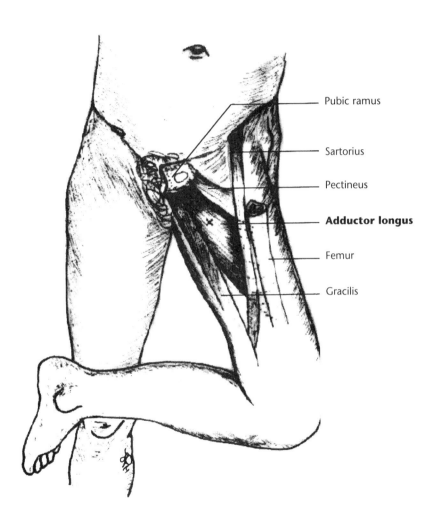

Pubic ramus

Sartorius

Pectineus

Adductor longus

Femur

Gracilis

71. Adductor Magnus

Patient position: Supine, both thighs spread apart (abducted), the testing thigh externally rotated, and the knee flexed

Needle insertion: In the above position, note the ischial tuberosity and gracilis muscle. Insert the needle approximately 10 cm distal to the anteromedial side of the ischial tuberosity and immediately medial to the gracilis.

Activation: The adductor magnus consists of anterior and posterior fibers.

Anterior fibers: Adduction and flexion of the thigh

Posterior fibers: Adduction and extension of the thigh

Clinical notes: Largest muscle of the adductor group. It is located deep. Functionally it has two groups: adductors and hamstring.

Innervation: Anterior part (fibers) L3, L4—obturator nerve (posterior division)

Posterior part (fibers)—L5, S1—tibial division of sciatic nerve

Origin (O) and Insertion (I):

Anterior Fibers
(O) Inferior ramus of the pubis, and ramus of the ischium
(I) Medial lip of the linea aspera of the femur

Posterior Fibers
(O) Ischial tuberosity
(I) Adductor tubercle of the medial epicondyle of the femur

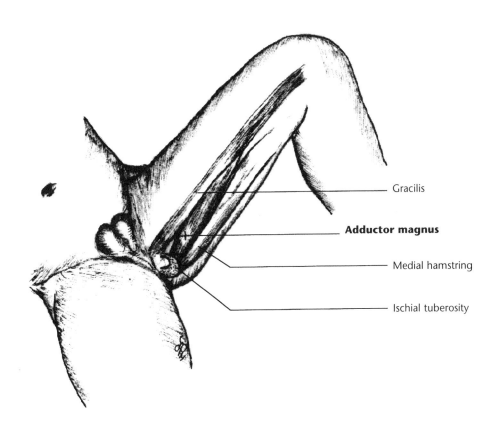

Gracilis

Adductor magnus

Medial hamstring

Ischial tuberosity

72. Gracilis

Patient position: Supine with the hip flexed, abducted, and externally rotated. The testing leg is placed over the opposite leg.

Needle insertion: In the above position, insert the needle at the proximal one-third of the most medial side of the thigh where a cordlike, tight muscle belly is palpable.

Activation: Raise the thigh against resistance from the above position (flexion and adduction of the hip).

Clinical notes: It is a superficial, thin, flat, straplike muscle located superficially on the medial side of the knee and thigh. It is the weakest muscle of the adductor group and the only one to cross the knee.

Innervation: L2, L3—obturator nerve (anterior division)

Origin: Inferior ramus of the pubis and ramus of the ischium

Insertion: Medial proximal end of tibia just distal to medial condyle

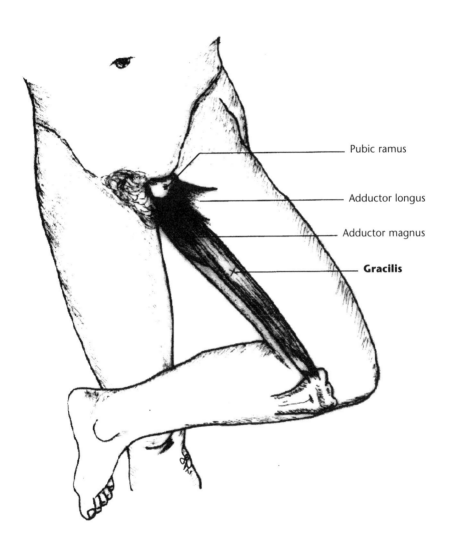

Pubic ramus

Adductor longus

Adductor magnus

Gracilis

THE BUTTOCK AND POSTERIOR THIGH

73. Gluteus Maximus

Patient position: Side-lying or prone

Needle insertion: From the upper end of the intergluteal cleft, insert the needle 2 to 3 cm down and the same distance laterally, but above the gluteal fold. The needle can also be inserted approximately 5 cm straight above the ischial tuberosity.

Activation: Extend the hip with the knee flexed. Ask the patient to squeeze his/her buttocks together.

Clinical notes: It is the largest and heaviest muscle in the body and is quadrilateral in shape. It is the most superficial muscle of the buttock region. It has three bursae, one that separates it from the greater trochanter of the femur, one from the vastus lateralis, and the other from the ischial tuberosity.

Examined for:

♦ S1, S2 radiculopathy
♦ Inferior gluteal neuropathy
♦ Unspecified leg pain

Innervation: L5, S1, and S2—inferior gluteal nerve

Origin: Posterior iliac crest, posterior superior iliac spine, posterior surface of the sacrotuberous ligament, dorsum of the sacrum and coccyx, and posterior portion of the sacroiliac ligament

Insertion: Gluteal tuberosity of the femur—(one-fourth to one-half of total fibers) Iliotibial band (tract) to the lateral condyle of the tibia—(one-half to three-fourths of total fibers)

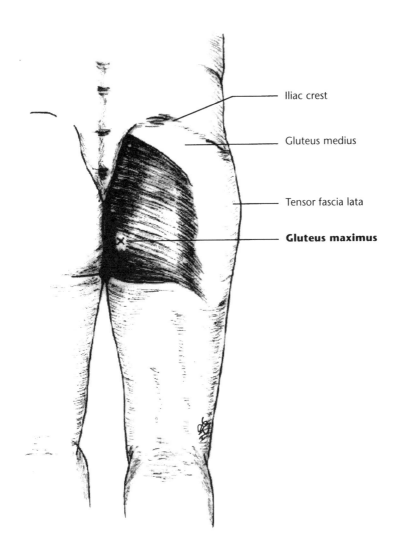

Iliac crest

Gluteus medius

Tensor fascia lata

Gluteus maximus

74. Gluteus Medius

Patient position: Side-lying or prone

Needle insertion: Note a line drawn between the iliac crest and greater trochanter of the femur. Insert the needle approximately 5 cm inferior from the iliac crest. If inserted too inferiorly and deeply, it will be in the gluteus minimus.

Activation: Abduct and internally rotate the thigh (leg)

Clinical notes: Broad, thick muscle on the outer surface of the pelvis. Its posterior portion lies deep to the gluteus maximus. It is the main hip abductor.

Examined for:

+ L5 radiculopathy
+ Superior gluteal neuropathy
+ Unspecified lower extremity pain

Innervation: L5 and S1—superior gluteal nerve

Origin: External one-half of the ilium and the iliac crest

Insertion: Greater trochanter of the femur

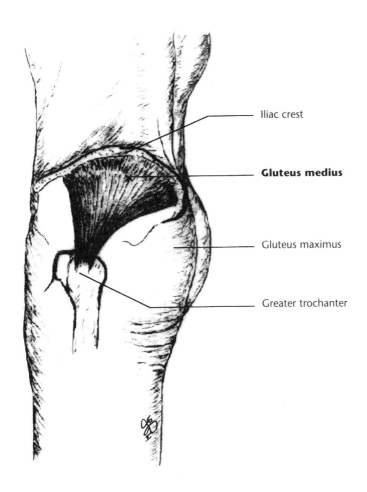

Iliac crest

Gluteus medius

Gluteus maximus

Greater trochanter

75. Gluteus Minimus

Patient position: Prone or lateral recumbent

Needle insertion: Insert the needle at approximately the midpoint of a line drawn between the greater trochanter of the femur and the iliac crest. This muscle is deep to the gluteus medius. Withdraw the needle a few millimeters to examine the muscle after it touches the iliac bone.

Activation: Abduct the hip.

Innervation: L5, S1—superior gluteal nerve

Clinical notes: Fan-shaped muscle that lies deep to the gluteus medius and is the smallest of the abductor group

Origin: Inferior lateral surface of the wing of the ilium between the anterior and inferior gluteal lines

Insertion: Greater trochanter of the femur

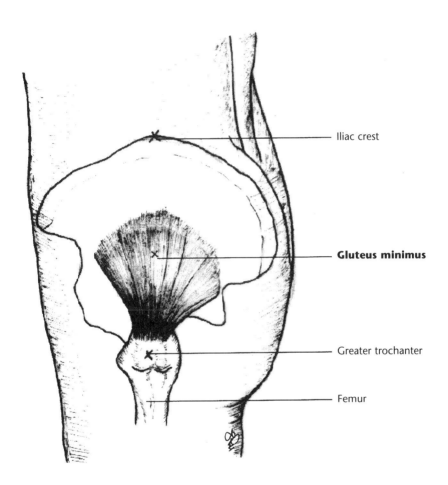

Iliac crest

Gluteus minimus

Greater trochanter

Femur

76. Piriformis

Patient position: Prone or side-lying

Needle insertion: Insert the needle at the junction of the upper and middle third of a line drawn between the greater trochanter and posterior inferior iliac spine (PIIS), or a few cm below the PIIS.

Activation: Lateral rotation of the extended thigh or abduction of the flexed thigh

Clinical notes: This muscle is deep to the gluteus maximus and almost parallel with the posterior margin of the gluteus medius. Its lower border (space between the piriformis and superior gemellus) is in contact with the sciatic nerve. It is frequently pierced by the common peroneal nerve, which is the lateral portion of the sciatic nerve.

Innervation: S1, S2—nerve to the piriformis

Origin: Anterior aspect of the second, third, and fourth sacral vertebrae and the sacrotuberous ligament

Insertion: Upper border of the greater trochanter of the femur

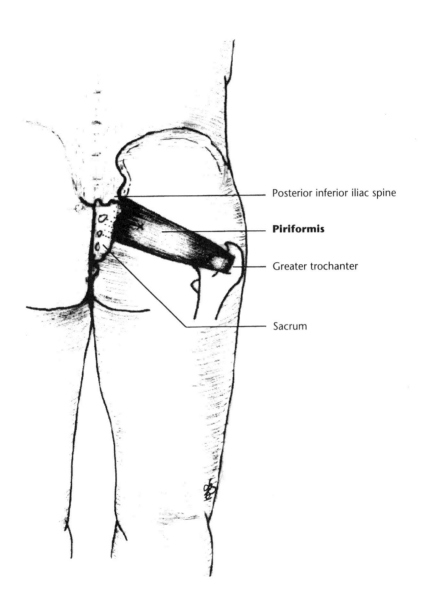

Posterior inferior iliac spine

Piriformis

Greater trochanter

Sacrum

77. Quadratus Femoris

Patient position: Lateral decubitus or prone

Needle insertion: Insert the needle at the midpoint of a line drawn between the ischial tuberosity and the greater trochanter of the femur.

Activation: Externally rotate the thigh.

Clinical notes: It is a flat, quadrilateral-shaped muscle that lies between the inferior gemellus and the upper margin of the adductor magnus.

Innervation: L5 and S1—nerve to quadratus femoris

Origin: Lateral aspect of the ischial tuberosity, immediately below the inferior gemellus

Insertion: Trochanteric crest of the femur

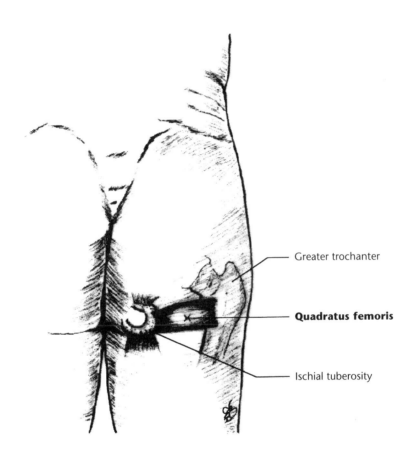

Greater trochanter

Quadratus femoris

Ischial tuberosity

78. Biceps Femoris—Long Head

Patient position: Prone or side-lying

Needle insertion: Insert the needle at the midpoint of a line drawn between the ischial tuberosity and tendon of the lateral hamstring at the popliteal fossa.

Activation: Extend the thigh with the leg flexed.

Clinical notes: The long and short heads of the biceps femoris forms the lateral hamstrings. If the needle is inserted too deeply close to the femur, it will be in the short head of the biceps femoris; too medially, in the medial hamstring (semimembranosus or semitendinosus).

Innervation: L5, S1, S2—sciatic nerve (tibial portion)

Origin: Ischial tuberosity (common tendon with the semitendinosus)

Insertion: Head of the fibula

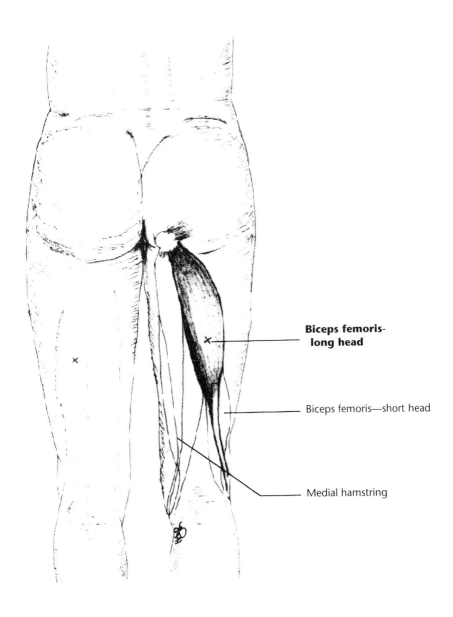

**Biceps femoris-
long head**

Biceps femoris—short head

Medial hamstring

79.   Biceps Femoris—Short Head

Patient position: Prone or side-lying

Needle insertion: Insert the needle immediately lateral or medial to the tendon of the biceps femoris—long head at the level of the popliteal fossa or above, and advance it toward the posterior aspect of the femur.

Activation: Flex the knee.

Clinical notes: The short head may be congenitally absent. It is the only thigh muscle innervated by the common peroneal nerve. Foot drop may be complicated by a lesion of a peripheral nerve, frequently the common peroneal nerve at the head of the fibula or the peroneal portion of the sciatic nerve in the thigh. In a patient with foot drop, this muscle should be examined to localize the nerve lesion at the fibula head or in the thigh.

Innervation: L5, S1—common peroneal portion of the sciatic nerve

Origin: Lateral lip of the entire linear aspera of the femur and the proximal lateral supracondylar line of the femur

Insertion: Head of the fibula

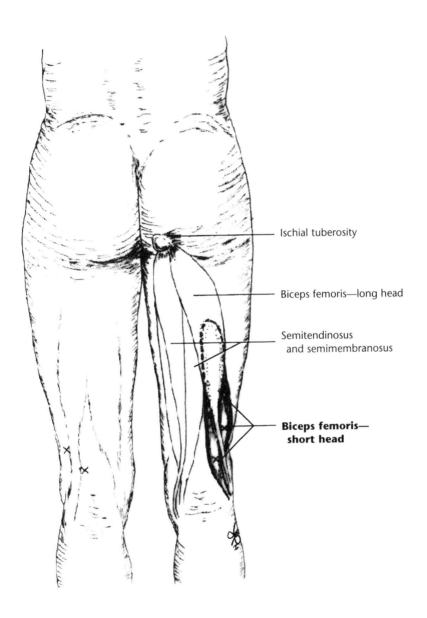

Ischial tuberosity

Biceps femoris—long head

Semitendinosus
and semimembranosus

**Biceps femoris—
short head**

The Buttock and Posterior Thigh   *175*

80. Semitendinosus

Patient position: Prone or side-lying

Needle insertion: Insert the needle midway between the ischial tuberosity and the medial hamstring tendons at the popliteal fossa.

Activation: Extend the thigh with the knee flexed.

Clinical notes: This muscle is fusiform in shape and is the most superficial of the hamstring group. Along with the semimembranosus and the hamstrings portion of the adductor magnus, forms the medial hamstrings. If the needle is inserted too laterally, it will be in the biceps femoris; too deeply, in the semimembranosus.

Activation: Flex the knee and extend the hip.

Innervation: L5, S1—tibial portion of the sciatic nerve

Origin: Ischial tuberosity, from a common tendon with the long head of the biceps femoris

Insertion: Medial surface of the upper tibia, posterior to the insertion of the sartorius and gracilis

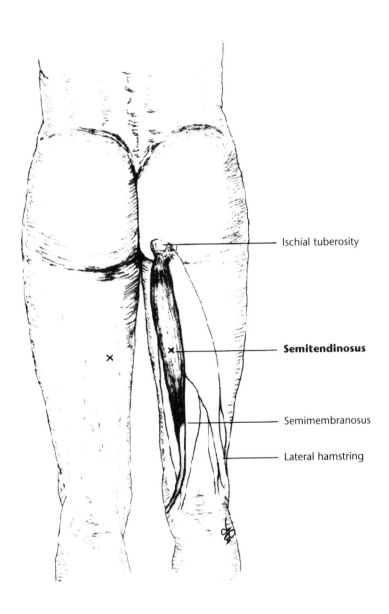

Ischial tuberosity

Semitendinosus

Semimembranosus

Lateral hamstring

The Buttock and Posterior Thigh *177*

81. Semimembranosus

Patient position: Prone or side-lying

Needle insertion: The needle is inserted immediately lateral to the tendon of the semitendinosus at the level of the popliteal fossa or above.

Clinical notes: The proximal half of this muscle is deep to the semitendinosus and the long head of the biceps femoris.

Activation: Flex and internally rotate the flexed knee and extend the hip.

Innervation: L5, S1, S2—tibial portion of the sciatic nerve

Origin: Ischial tuberosity

Insertion: Posteromedial aspect of the medial tibial condyle. A heavy band comes off the site of the insertion and runs obliquely upward and laterally, blending with the posterior capsule of the knee joint to form the oblique popliteal ligament, which inserts into the soleal line of the posterior tibia.

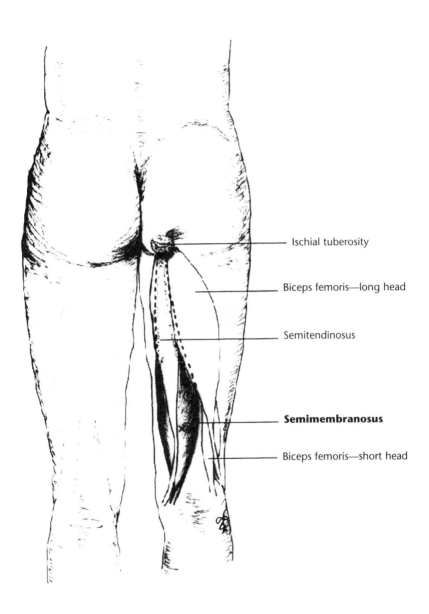

Ischial tuberosity

Biceps femoris—long head

Semitendinosus

Semimembranosus

Biceps femoris—short head

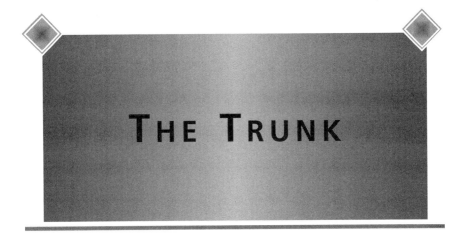

THE TRUNK

82. Diaphragm

Patient position: Supine

Needle insertion: **Bolton's method:** One of several interspaces between the medial clavicular and anterior axillary lines in the lower costal margins. A monopolar needle is inserted just above the costal margin at a right angle to the chest wall. As the needle advances, recordings can be made through the muscles of chest wall (e.g., external oblique or rectus abdominis, external and internal costal muscles) and then, finally, the diaphragm.

(*Reference:* Bolton CF: AAEM Minimonography #40: Clinical Neurophysiology of the respiratory system. *Muscle & Nerve* 16: 809–818, 1993)

Saadeh et al. method: The needle is inserted at the point where the paramidclavicular line (the line drawn at the halfway between the jugular notch of the sternum and the lateral border of the clavicle) intersects the lower costal margin at the ninth rib cartilage. The needle slowly advances through the skin and abdominal muscle, and closely hugging the posterior aspect of the chest wall, while the examiner's free hand depresses the abdominal wall. A 50 mm long of monopolar needle is recommended.

(*Reference:* Saadeh PB, Crisafulli CF, Bosner J, Wolf E: Needle electromyography of the diaphragm: A new technique. *Muscle & Nerve* 16: 15–20, 1993)

Activation: Regular breathing

Clinical notes: Potential complications: pneumothorax, pneumoperitonium, bleeding. Examined for:

♦ C3, C4 radiculopathy
♦ Phrenic neuropathy

Contraindication: Severe obesity, marked abdominal distension.

Innervation: C3, C4, C5—phrenic nerve (right and left)

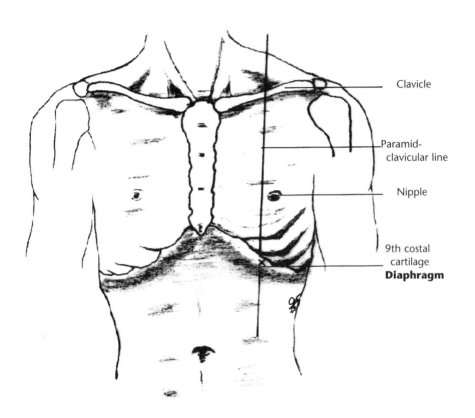

Clavicle

Paramid-clavicular line

Nipple

9th costal cartilage
Diaphragm

Saadeh et al. method

82. Diaphragm (*continued*)

Origin:

1. Sternal part—posterior surface of the xyphoid process

2. Costal part—inner internal surface of the anterior ends of costal cartilages 7 through 12

3. Lateral arcuate ligament—from the twelfth rib to the transverse process of first lumbar vertebrae bilaterally

4. Medial arcuate ligament—from the transverse process of the first lumbar vertebrae and the body of the second lumbar vertebrae bilaterally

5. Lumbar part—arises from the two fibrous arches (medial and lateral arcuate ligament) and the bodies of lumbar vertebrae two and three

Insertion:

Inserts upon itself in a central tendon

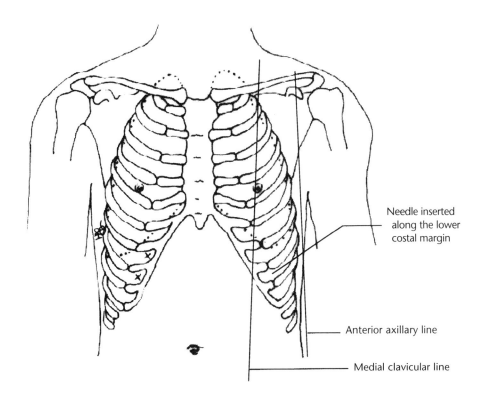

Needle inserted along the lower costal margin

Anterior axillary line

Medial clavicular line

Bolton's method

83. Intercostalis—External and Internal

Patient position: Supine or lateral recumbent

Needle insertion: Spaces between the midclavicular and anterior axillary line at the seventh or eighth intercostal space. The needle is inserted along the upper margin of the rib tangentially at a relatively sharp angle. Before the insertion, spread the intercostal spaces out by full flexion of the arm.

Activation: Ask the patient to inspire deeply.

Innervation: T1–T11—intercostal nerves

Origin: Lower border of the rib above

Insertion: Upper border of the rib below the origin

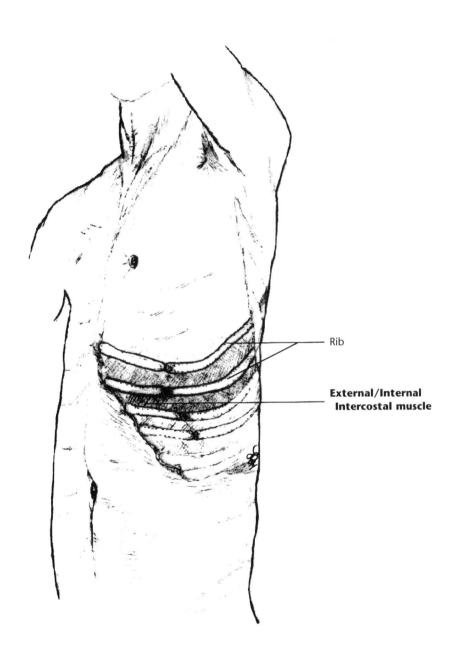

Rib

External/Internal
Intercostal muscle

84. Rectus Abdominis

Patient position: Supine

Needle insertion: Insert the needle transversely from near the midclavicular line (or linea semilunaris) toward the linea alba in the abdominal wall. Depending on the thickness of the subcutaneous fat, it may need a few cm insertion of the needle electrode to reach the muscle from the skin.

Clinical notes: Long, straplike muscles that extend the whole length of the front of the abdomen. These are paired muscles separated by the linea alba that lie under the anterior layer of the rectus sheet.

Examined for:

◆ Lower thoracic radiculopathy

◆ Lower intercostal neuropathy

Activation: Trunk flexion

Innervation: T6 (T5)–T12—ventral rami of the lower six thoracic nerves (intercostals)

Origin: Pubic symphysis, and pubic crest

Insertion: Fifth, sixth, seventh costal cartilages, and the anterior aspect of the xyphoid process

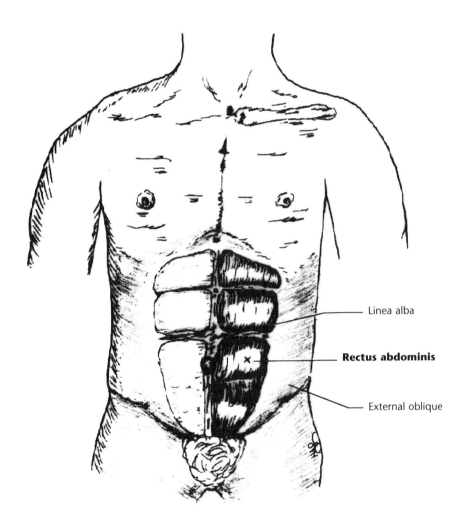

Linea alba

Rectus abdominis

External oblique

85. External Oblique (Obliquus Externus Abdominis)

Patient position: Supine or lateral decubitus

Needle insertion: The needle is introduced in a space between the midclavicular and anterior axillary lines in the abdomen or intercostal spaces (seventh rib or below).

Clinical notes: Paired muscles that are the largest and most superficial of the anterior abdominal wall muscles. This is a broad, thin muscle that curves around the lateral and anterior part of the abdomen.

Examined for:

◆ Thoracic radiculopathy
◆ Isolated intercostal neuropathy

Activation: Flex and rotate the trunk along with the internal oblique.

Innervation: Ventral rami of the lower six thoracic spinal nerves (intercostals)

Origin: Anterior surface of the lower six ribs (external surface and inferior border of each rib)

Insertion: Anterior part of iliac crest, tendinous extension to the anterior superior iliac spine and the pubic tubercle and crest

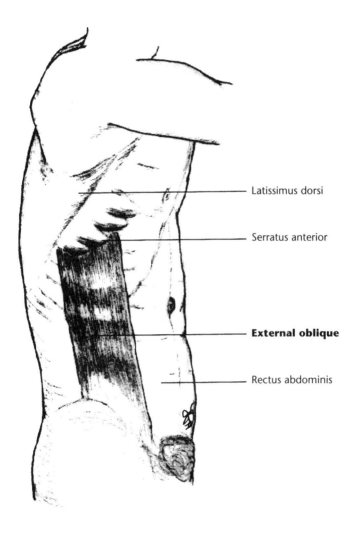

Latissimus dorsi

Serratus anterior

External oblique

Rectus abdominis

86-1. Cervical Paraspinal Muscles/Multifidi

Patient position: Lateral decubitus with neck fully flexed. The neck is comfortably supported with a pillow. This position preferable to the prone position.

Needle insertion: Note the most prominent spinous process (C7) with the neck fully flexed. At approximately 2 to 3 cm lateral to the spinous process, the needle advances directly toward the transverse process until it strikes the transverse process and is withdrawn a bit and redirected toward the groove to check the multifidus.

Activation: Ask the patient to extend his/her neck gently while checking motor unit activities.

Clinical notes: These fibers are short and oblique bundles that are the strongest in the cervical and lumbar regions. Examined for:

♦ Cervical radiculopathy

♦ Differential diagnosis of brachial plexopathy vs cervical radiculopathy

♦ Localized paraspinal lesions etc.

Innervation: Cervical dorsal rami of the corresponding spinal nerves

Origin and Insertion: Transverse processes to spinous processes, the muscle fascicles are obliquely placed (fibers run upward and medially) in relation to the vertebral column and extend two to four segments in length.

(Neck fully flexed)

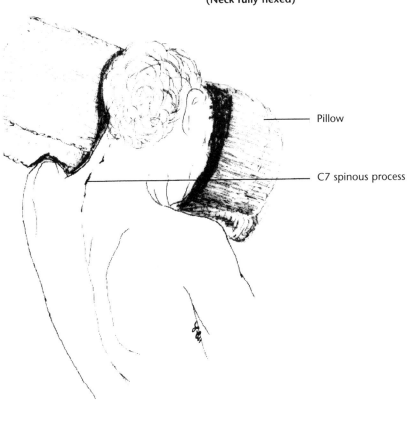

Pillow

C7 spinous process

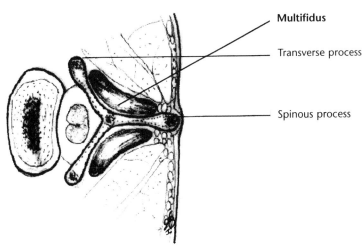

Multifidus

Transverse process

Spinous process

86-2.   Lumbosacral Paraspinal Muscles/Multifidi

Patient position: Lateral decubitus with hip and knee fully flexed (fetal or scoop position) or prone position.

Needle insertion: Note the anatomic landmarks—posterior superior and inferior iliac spines, lumbar spinous processes and upper sacral spinous process, iliac crest, L5 and S1 interdisc space. Insert the needle approximately 3 or 4 cm lateral to the spinous process and advance it straight down until it reaches the transverse process. The needle is then withdrawn a bit and redirected toward the groove to check the multifidus.

Activation: Ask the patient to extend upper body or trunk a little bit.

Clinical notes: Examined for:

♦ Lumbosacral radiculopathy

♦ Localized paraspinal lesions

Innervation: Lumbosacral dorsal lami of the corresponding spinal nerves

Origin and Insertion: Transverse processes to spinous processes, the muscle fascicles are obliquely placed (fibers run upward and medially) in relation to the vertebral column and extend two to four segments in length.

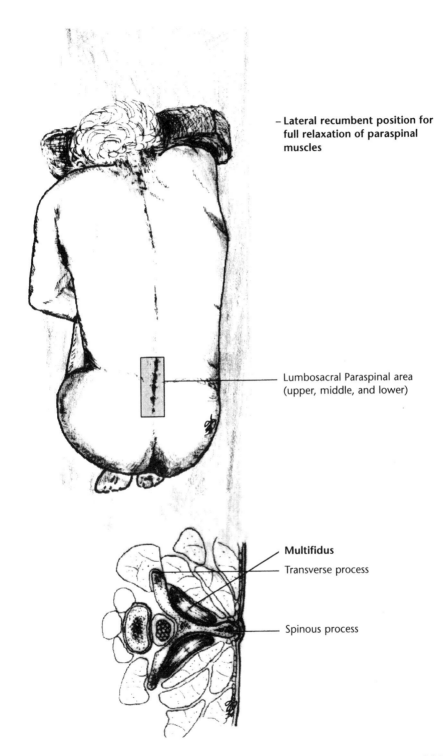

– Lateral recumbent position for full relaxation of paraspinal muscles

Lumbosacral Paraspinal area (upper, middle, and lower)

Multifidus

Transverse process

Spinous process

THE PELVIS

87.　External Anal Sphincter

Patient position:　Side-lying on the opposite side or supine

Needle insertion:　Insert the gloved index finger into the rectum to guide the direction of needle into the external anal sphincter. Insert the needle parallel to the inserted finger at the junction between the mucosal membrane and skin of the external anal sphincter (mucocutaneous junction). Prefer to insert the needle at the direction of the 6 o'clock or 9 o'clock position.

Activation:　Ask the patient to squeeze examiner's inserted gloved finger or ask the patient to act as during defecation to obtain relaxation.

Clinical notes:　It encircles the anal orifice. This muscle is often tested in lesions of the cauda equina or conus medullaris including the pudendal nerve and S2, S3, and S4. It may also be innervated by a perineal branch of sacral nerve 4.

Innervation:　S2, S3, S4—sacral plexus—pudendal nerve (branch called the inferior rectal nerve)

Origin:　Apex of coccyx and anococcygeal raphe

Insertion:　Muscle fibers decussate around the anus and meet anteriorly at the central point of perineum (central tendon of the perineum in front and the coccyx behind) and the deep surface of the skin.

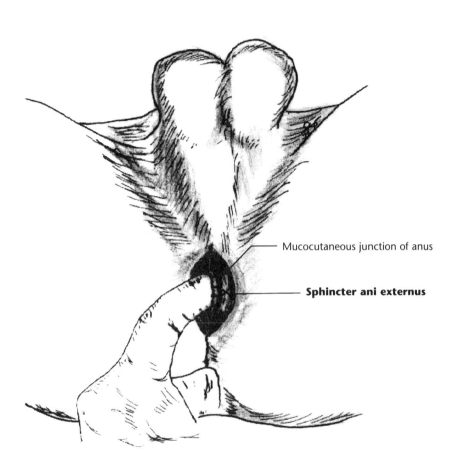

Mucocutaneous junction of anus

Sphincter ani externus

88. Bulbocavernosus (Bulbospongiosus)

Patient position: Supine, hip flexed and abducted (thigh spread apart), knee flexed

Needle insertion: It is a superficial, small, and thin layer of muscle. It is preferable to use a small needle electrode.

Male: Approximately midway between the root of penis (corpus spongiosum penis) and anus, a few millimeters lateral to the median line of the perineum. Using a very short needle, insert it at a sharp angle vertically.

Female: Immediately lateral to the labium minus (between labium minus and majus) at the level of the posterior labial commissure

Activation: Ask the patient to tighten all perineal and thigh muscles (as if to arrest defecation).

Innervation: S2, S3, S4—pudendal nerve (perineal branch)

Origin: In male, median raphe of the bulb of the penis and the perineal body; in female, surrounds the orifice of the vagina.

Insertion: **Male:** Upper surface of corpus spongiosum penis

Female: Corpora cavernosa clitoridis

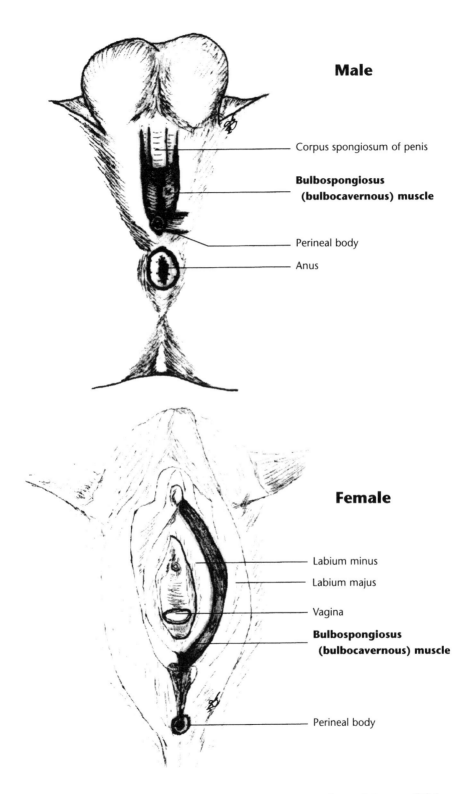

Male

Corpus spongiosum of penis

Bulbospongiosus (bulbocavernous) muscle

Perineal body

Anus

Female

Labium minus

Labium majus

Vagina

Bulbospongiosus (bulbocavernous) muscle

Perineal body

THE HEAD AND NECK

89. Frontalis

Patient position: Supine with head slightly turned (tilted) to the opposite side.

Needle insertion: The muscle is flat and extremely thin. Insert a short and small needle into the muscle at a 10 to 20 degree angle to the skin (relatively sharp angle) approximately at the midpoint between the front hairline and the eyebrow.

Activation: Ask the patient to raise the eyebrows or wrinkle the forehead.

Clinical notes: It has no bony attachments. Examined for:

+ Facial neuropathy (injury)
+ Single fiber electromyography

Normal MUAP amplitude and duration in this muscle are usually small and short. It is often difficult to differentiate from fibrillation potentials. It also fires rapidly.

Innervation: Facial nerve (C-VII)

Origin and Insertion: From the galea aponeurotica and ends in neighboring muscles and in the skin at the root of the nose and along the eyebrows

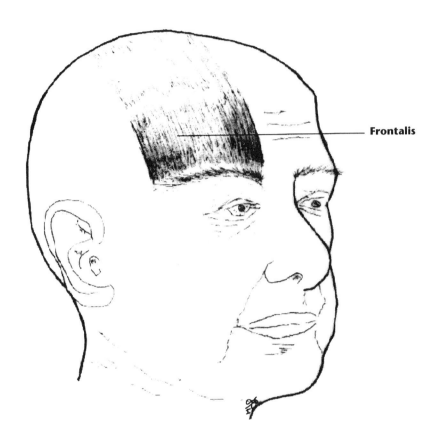

Frontalis

90. Orbicularis Oculi

Patient position: Supine with head slightly tilted to the opposite side

Needle insertion: Before inserting the needle, make sure of the orbital fossa and its lateral, upper, and inferior borders. Insert the needle approximately 1.5 cm from the lateral bony margin of the orbital fossa and direct it upward or downward obliquely. Insert and advance the needle at a relatively sharp angle because the muscle layer is extremely thin and superficial.

Activation: Close eyelids.

Clinical notes: It is a thin, flat, elliptical sphincter that surrounds the rim of the orbit. Important muscle from a cosmetic (facial expression) and functional (eye closure) standpoint after facial paralysis. "Black and blue markings" may result from needling. A firm compression with dry cotton or gauze may be necessary after the needle is removed. Examined for:

  ♦ Facial nerve injury
  ♦ Single Fiber EMG

Innervation: Facial nerve (C-VII)

Origin: Nasal part of the frontal bone, frontal process of the maxilla and anterior surface of the medial palpebral ligament

Insertion: Muscle fibers surround the circumference of the orbit, spread downward on the check, and blend with adjacent structures.

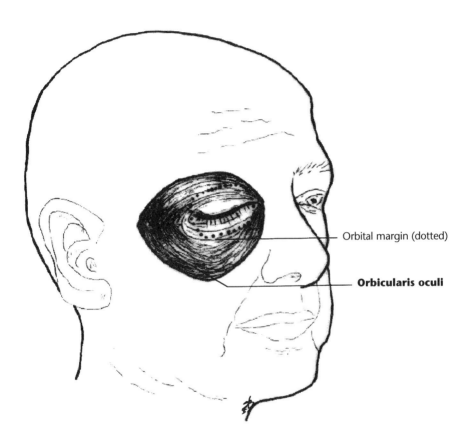

Orbital margin (dotted)

Orbicularis oculi

91. Orbicularis Oris

Patient position: Supine with the head slightly tilted to opposite side

Needle insertion: Insert the needle approximately 0.5 to 1 cm below or above the mouth angle and gradually advance it toward the midline while having the patient pucker his/her lips.

Activation: Ask the patient to whistle or pucker the lips.

Clinical notes: Examined for facial neuropathy. Very important muscle for facial expression or functional concerns after facial paralysis. Rare, but isolated neuropathy of superior or inferior buccal branches of facial nerve may be seen. Therefore, both upper and lower parts of this muscle may need to be tested separately.

Innervation: Facial nerve (C-VII)

Origin: Numerous strata of muscle fibers surrounding the orifice of the mouth, derived in part from other facial muscles such as the buccinator

Insertion: External skin and mucous membrane

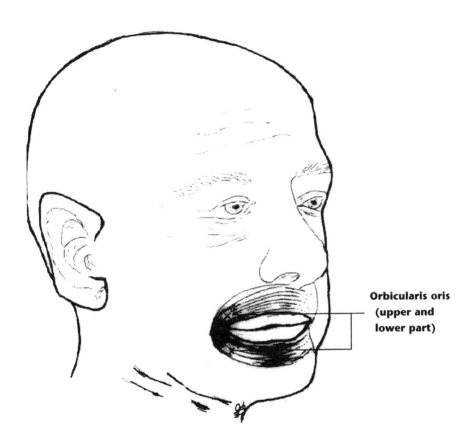

Orbicularis oris
(upper and
lower part)

92. Nasalis

Patient position:	Supine and head tilted slightly to the opposite side
Needle insertion:	Approximately 0.5 cm down from the ridge of nose, insert the needle parallel to the mid-portion of the side wall of the nostril toward the root of the nose. This muscle is extremely thin and superficial. Insert a very small needle at a sharp angle.
Activation:	Widen the aperture of the nostril either by deep inspiration through the nose or by force expiration through one nostril while compressing shut the other with a finger.
Clinical notes:	Examined for:

♦ Facial neuropathy

♦ Recording the compound muscle action potential in facial nerve conduction study. Probably less important clinically or functionally than orbicularis oris or orbicularis oculi.

Innervation:	Facial nerve (C-VII)
Origin:	Maxilla
Insertion:	Ala of the nose and aponeurosis of the opposite side of the nasalis

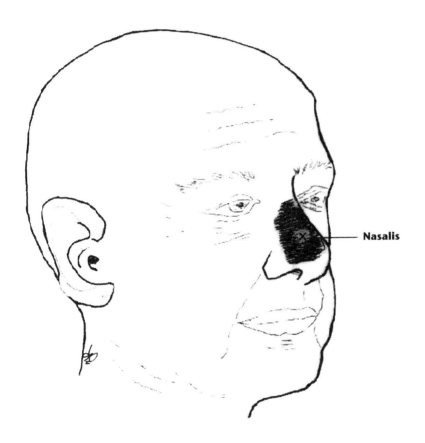

Nasalis

93. Mentalis

Patient position: Supine with the chin up

Needle insertion: Insert the needle approximately 0.5 to 1 cm lateral to the midline of the chin and from the lower border of the mandible. Advance it gradually upward.

Activation: Ask the patient to raise and protrude his/her lower lip.

Innervation: Marginal branch of the mandibular nerve of the facial nerve (C-VII)

Origin: Incisive fossa of the mandible

Insertion: Skin of the chin

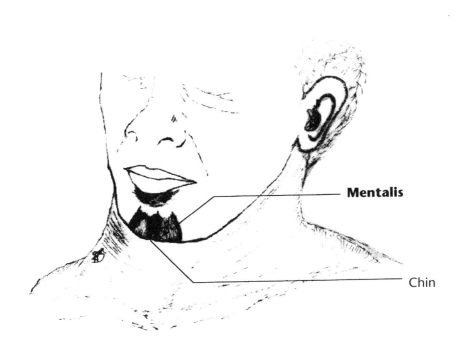

Mentalis

Chin

94. Auricularis Posterior

Patient position: Supine with the head turned to the opposite side of the examination, or side-lying, or sitting

Needle insertion: This muscle is superficial and extremely thin. By pulling the ear forward, a fold is made at the mid-portion of the posterior aspect of the pinna. The needle is inserted into the fold (muscle under skin crease). A voluntary contraction is very difficult but you may observe the motor unit action potentials by pulling the ear lobe forward or backward.

Clinical notes: This muscle may be normal if facial neuropathy may result from a lesion distal to the styloid foramen (e.g., parotid gland abscess).

Innervation: Facial nerve (C-VII)

Origin: Mastoid portion of the temporal bone

Insertion: Ponticulus on the eminentia conchae of the auricle

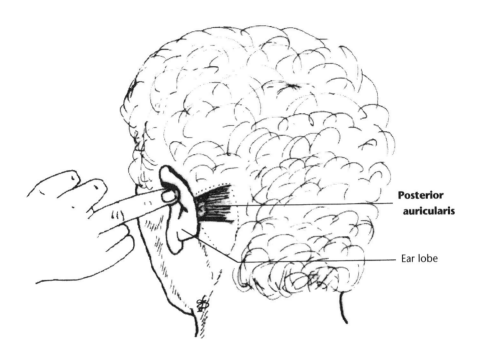

Posterior
auricularis

Ear lobe

95. Temporalis

Patient position: Supine with the head turned to the opposite side

Needle insertion: The muscle is thin and superficial. Insert a small needle at the level of eyebrow and advance it toward the temporal area at a relatively sharp angle to the skin (10 to 20 degrees).

Activation: Ask the subject to clench his/her teeth.

Clinical notes: It is a fan-shaped muscle that lies in the temporal fossa. Examined for trigeminal neuropathy (mandibular division)

Innervation: Trigeminal nerve (C-V)—deep temporal branches of the anterior trunk of the mandibular nerve

Origin: Floor of the temporal fossa and the temporal fascia

Insertion: Coronoid process and anterior border of the ramus of the mandible

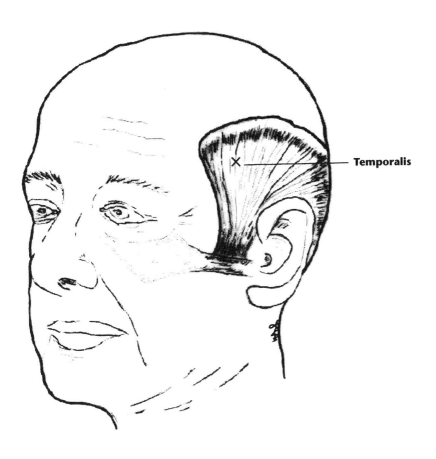

Temporalis

96. Masseter

Patient position: Supine and with the head turned to the opposite side

Needle insertion: Note the ramus of mandible and its jaw angle. In order to palpate this muscle bulk near the jaw angle, ask the subject to clench his/her teeth. Insert the needle over the muscle belly near the jaw angle or at the midpoint between the zygomatic arch and angle of the mandible.

Activation: Clench his/her teeth.

Clinical notes: Examined for trigeminal neuropathy. Avoid injury to the parotid gland that is located near the ear lobe and the mandibular angle area.

Innervation: Trigeminal nerve (C-V)—a branch of the anterior trunk of the mandibular nerve

Origin: Zygomatic process of the maxilla and anterior two-thirds of zygomatic arch

Insertion: Lateral surface of the ramus and angle of the mandible

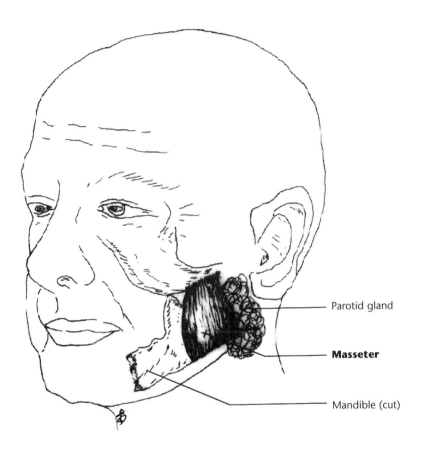

Parotid gland

Masseter

Mandible (cut)

97. Cricothyroid

Patient position: Supine with the head in midline and the neck in slight extension.

Needle insertion: The needle is inserted at the level of the superior border and just off the midline of the cricoid cartilage. The needle is directed superiorly and laterally toward the thyroid cartilage while the patient is vocalizing.

Clinical notes: Most superficial of the laryngeal muscles. Make sure of the anatomic landmarks (e.g., thyroid cartilage, cricoid cartilage) before inserting the needle. The muscle is so thin that it requires a very small and short electrode to perform the test. Phonation is necessary to activate the motor units.

Innervation: Superior laryngeal nerve (external laryngeal branch), which is a branch of the vagus nerve (C-X).

Origin: Front and lateral parts of the outer surface of the cricoid cartilage

Insertion: Posterior part of the lower border of the lamina of the thyroid cartilage and into the anterior border of the inferior horn

(*Reference:* Rodriquez AA, Simpson DM: 1996 AAEM Course E: Approach to the patient with bulbar symptoms—Case illustrations.)

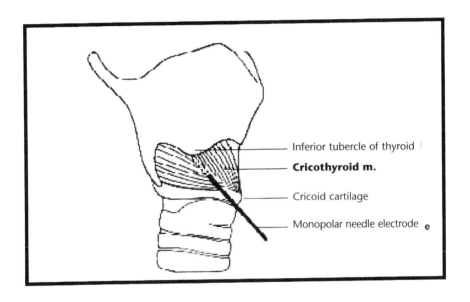

Inferior tubercle of thyroid

Cricothyroid m.

Cricoid cartilage

Monopolar needle electrode e

98. Thyroarytenoid

Patient position: Supine, neck in slight extension and the head in midline

Needle insertion

and Activation: A small, short needle is inserted just superior to the cricoid cartilage in the midline and directed: superiorly, 70 degrees; laterally, 15 degrees. The needle is advancing deep to the thyroid cartilage while the patient vocalizes a high-pitched "E."

Innervation: Recurrent laryngeal nerve, branch of the vagus nerve (C-X)

Origin: Medial surface of the lamina of the thyroid cartilage, and the cricothyroid ligament.

Insertion: Anterolateral surface of the arytenoid cartilage

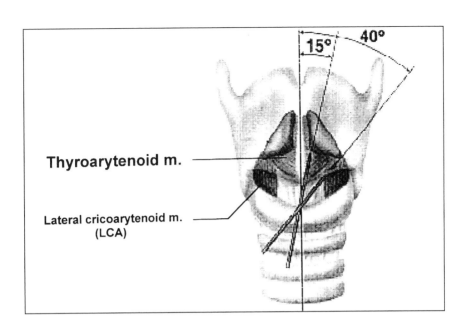

Thyroarytenoid m.

Lateral cricoarytenoid m.
(LCA)

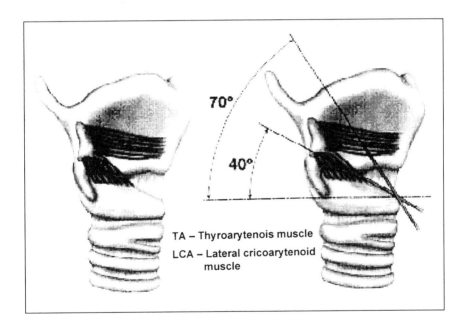

TA – Thyroarytenois muscle
LCA – Lateral cricoarytenoid
muscle

99. Sternocleidomastoid

Patient position: Supine

Needle insertion: Palpate the mid-portion of muscle belly, while rotating head to side opposite, or while flexing head to the same shoulder. Hold the medial and lateral borders of muscle belly by the thumb and index fingers at the mid-portion and insert the needle.

Activation: Tilt the head toward the shoulder of the same side, or rotate the head toward the opposite side.

Clinical notes: Examined for accessory neuropathy, often occurring after radical neck dissection. Advance the needle with care because there are many neurovascular structures under this muscle.

Innervation: Accessory nerve (C-XI) C2, C3, (ventral rami)

Origin: Front of the manubrium of the sternum and the upper surface of the medial one-third of the clavicle

Insertion: Lateral surface of the mastoid process and lateral one-half of the superior nuchal line of the occipital bone.

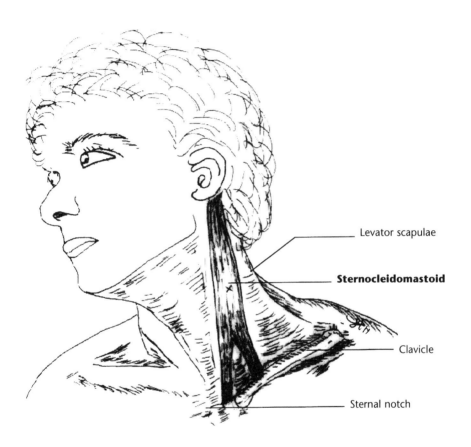

Levator scapulae

Sternocleidomastoid

Clavicle

Sternal notch

100. Tongue

Patient position: Supine with the head in the midline position and the neck in slight extension

Needle insertion:

1. The examiner's gloved fingers hold the patient's tongue after asking the patient to stick out his/her tongue. The needle is inserted on the side of the tongue.

2. Head is in extension. A needle is inserted 2 to 3 cm lateral to the tip of the chin laterally and just off the inner side of mandibular bone. The needle should pass through the mylohyoid and geniohyoid muscles to reach the tongue, genioglossus.

Activation: Ask the patient to stick his/her tongue out (protrude its apex from the mouth).

Clinical notes: The genioglossus is a fan-shaped muscle placed vertically that is in contact with its fellow medially. It makes up the bulk of the posterior tongue. Usually performed in search of possible motor neuron disease, amyotrophic lateral sclerosis

Innervation: Hypoglossal nerve (C-XII)

Origin: Genioglossus muscle: Upper genial tubercle on the inner surface of the symphysis of the mandible

Insertion: Inferior aspect of the tongue and into the front of the body of the hyoid bone.

Approach from the side wall of tongue

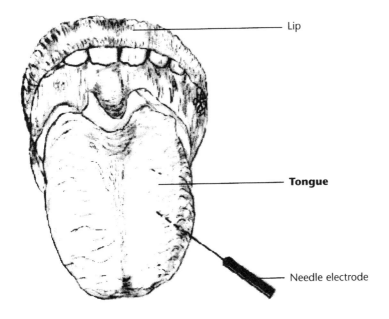

Lip

Tongue

Needle electrode

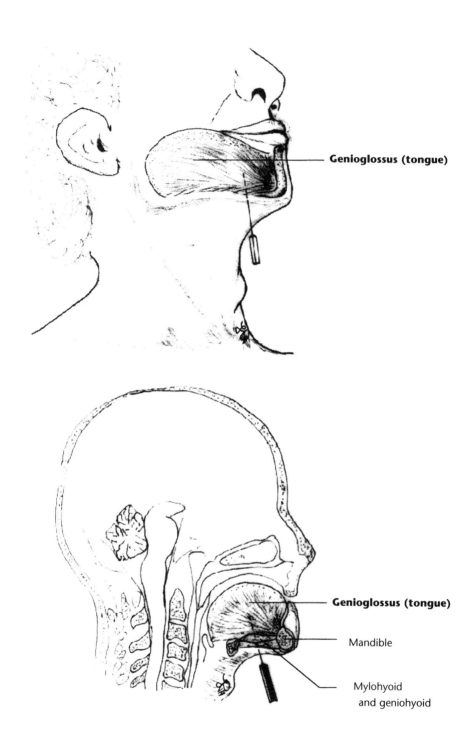

Genioglossus (tongue)

Genioglossus (tongue)

Mandible

Mylohyoid
and geniohyoid

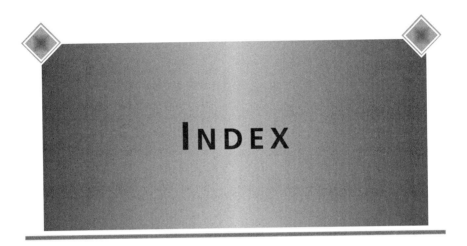

INDEX